Introduction
to Regional
Anaesthesia

Introduction to Regional Anaesthesia

D. BRUCE SCOTT

M.D., F.R.C.P.E., F.F.A.R.C.S.
Consultant Anaesthetist,
Royal Infirmary; and
Senior Lecturer,
Department of Anaesthetics,
University of Edinburgh,
Edinburgh, Scotland

LENNART HÅKANSSON

Coordinator

POUL BUCKHÖJ

Medical artist

Foreword by
MICHAEL ROSEN

M.D., F.F.A.R.C.S.
Department of Anaesthetics
University of Wales
Cardiff, Wales

APPLETON & LANGE/MEDIGLOBE
Norwalk, Connecticut/San Mateo, California/Fribourg, Switzerland

0-8385-4390-1

Notice: Our knowledge in clinical sciences is constantly changing. As new information becomes available, changes in treatment and in the use of drugs become necessary. The author(s) and the publisher of this volume have taken care to make certain that the doses of drugs and schedules of treatment are correct and compatible with the standards generally accepted at the time of publication. The reader is advised to consult carefully the instruction and information material included in the package insert of each drug or therapeutic agent before administration. This advice is especially important when using new or infrequently used drugs.

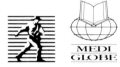

Prentice-Hall of Australia, Pty.Ltd., Sydney
Prentice-Hall Canada, Inc.
Prentice-Hall Hispanoamericana, S.A., Mexico
Prentice-Hall or India Private Limited, New Delhi
Prentice-Hall of Japan, Inc., Tokyo
Prentice-Hall of Southeast Asia (Pte.) Ltd., Singapore
Whitehall Books Ltd., Wellington, New Zealand
Editora Prentice-Hall do Brasil Ltda., Rio de Janeiro

Produced by
PACIFIC PRINT PRODUCTION AB
SWEDEN

Printed by
KIN KEONG PRINTING CO PTE LTD
SINGAPORE

Library of Congress Cataloging-in-Publication Data

Scott, D. Bruce (Donald Bruce)
    Introduction to regional anaesthesia.

Includes indes.
1. Conduction anesthesia. I Title. (DNLM:
1. Anesthesia, Conduction-methods. WO
300 S425i)
RD84.S47 1989
617'.964   89-10374

ISBN 0-8385-4390-1

Foreword

Then the eyes of those who see will not be closed and the ears of those who hear will hearken - Isiah 32;3

Currently there is a new realization that regional anaesthesia has an essential role to play in high quality anaesthetic practice and, especially in the control of postoperative pain. General, with local, anaesthesia can offer an elegant combination in which the patient benefits during surgery and has a pain-free recovery.

It is necessary to organise the theatre efficiently so as to accomplish these aims, which, then, need not make higher demands on time during the operating schedule. It is also essential to become familiar with common techniques of regional block during training and to renew knowledge of those perhaps subject to disuse atrophy. Dr. Scott has spent a lifetime as a leading teacher and researcher into the benefits of regional anaesthesia. His controlled enthusiasm and experience shine through the book. He has chosen to illustrate regional blocks which are most valuable; and to do so in perfect detail. There are no redandant statements, but each description gives all the answers to that essential question, "How to do it"?, which has eluded so many others. The illustrations are a perfect accompaniment to the text - which we might expect from that other master - Poul Buckhöj.

This book will encourage many to broaden their horizons, and to refresh their memories. It can only be to great benefit of our patients if every anaesthetist is encouraged to read (and to hear) about the many benefits that regional anaesthetic techniques can confer. This book should ensure that they do so.

Michael Rosen

Preface

There is now a consensus view that regional anaesthesia is an important part of the anaesthetist's armamentarium both for surgical anaesthesia and for pain control. As regional anaesthesia becomes more popular, an increasing portion of training programmes is being devoted to it.

In learning regional anaesthetic techniques, there is no substitute for personal tuition from an experienced practitioner. Nevertheless a knowledge of anatomy, pharmacology and toxicology is necessary if the trainee is to have a proper understanding of what he or she is being taught.

There is room for discussion regarding the number and variety of techniques which the practising anaesthetist should be capable of performing. This will depend primarily on the scope of the work being undertaken by the individual. For the purposes of this book a limited, but reasonably comprehensive, list of techniques has been chosen. Experience with these methods would form a solid base for trainees, some of whom might eventually wish to expand their repertoire.

Preliminary remarks are included on the pharmacology and toxicology, together with the general background knowledge regarding regional anaesthesia. It is hoped that the drawings give a clear picture of the anatomy. Instructions on how to perform each procedure have been given as simply as possible. They may indeed appear somewhat repetitive, but many readers will consult the text intermittently for specific nerve blocks, rather than read it from cover to cover.

There is seldom only one way of performing any anaesthetic procedure and this also applies to regional anaesthesia. I have described techniques which I have found to be effective and have eschewed offering a variety of alternatives. However all three of the common methods of brachial plexus block have been included as the choice is affected by both the surgical procedure and the patient.

I am indebted to many colleagues for their advice and help, particularly Poul Buckhöj for the outstanding drawings, Lennart Håkansson for the preparation and design and Pam Hindshaw for many hours of typing and correcting.

D.B. Scott

Contents

Introduction

Use of local or regional anaesthesia

Local or regional anaesthesia may be used for surgical procedures, for relief of acute or chronic pain, and for therapeutic or diagnostic purposes.

Advantages

The ability to render a specific part of the body anaesthetic without affecting the brain has many advantages, including:

1. The ability to have the patient conscious during surgery. Thus the patient can maintain his own airway and the inhalation of gastric contents is unlikely. For minor procedures, the presence of an anaesthetist is unnecessary.

2. A smooth recovery. Unlike general anaesthesia, many procedures do not require the same degree of nursing care that is necessary with an unconscious patient. Because in most cases local anaesthesia will still be present at the end of surgery, the patient will be awake and rational when pain eventually appears. This contrasts with the restlessness frequently seen in the semiconscious patient with severe pain after general anaesthesia.

3. Postoperative analgesia. In many instances it is possible to continue the local anaesthesia for hours or days, e.g. by using a catheter technique.

4. Reduction in surgical stress. The elimination of painful afferent stimuli from the operative site, plus the blockade of efferent sympathetic nerves to endocrine glands, eliminates or greatly reduces the metabolic and endocrine changes seen after surgical operations. This applies in the main to lower abdominal, perineal and limb surgery. The modification of surgical stress will be greatest when the local anaesthesia is continued for 1-2 days postoperatively.

5. Earlier discharge for outpatients or day patients.

6. Less expense.

Disadvantages

1. The patient may prefer to be asleep. This does not preclude the use of regional anaesthesia, which can be combined with a light general anaesthetic.

2. A degree of practice and skill is required for the best results. Operations on awake patients also involve the cooperation of the whole surgical team.

3. Some blocks require up to 30 min or more to be fully effective.

4. Analgesia may not always be totally effective. Thus the patient may require additional analgesics, or a light general anaesthetic.

5. Generalised toxicity may occur if the local anaesthetic drug is given intravenously by mistake, or an overdose is injected.

6. Some operations, e.g. thoracotomies, are unsuitable for local anaesthesia.

7. Widespread sympathetic blockade with resulting hypotension can occur with certain techniques, e.g. spinal or epidural blockade.

8. There is a small but definite incidence of prolonged nerve damage.

Preoperative assessment and preparation

The preoperative assessment of patients is not different from that required for general anaesthesia. Thus it is necessary to determine the general physical condition, to identify any relevant pathology and to assess the patient's attitude to the proposed anaesthetic technique.

The need to perform surgery using local or regional anaesthesia may vary from "mandatory" to "contraindicated" depending on circumstances. Thus a patient with an airway which cannot be guaranteed during general anaesthesia and who may be at risk from inhalation of gastric contents, requires to be awake during surgery. A patient with a strong desire to be awake, e.g. for the performance of a Caesarean section, will consider regional anaesthesia highly desirable. In other patients, widespread sympathetic blockade may be an unacceptable risk, e.g. those with uncorrected hypovolaemia.

Many patients may be unwilling at first to accept a local/regional anaesthetic. However, a proper explanation of the risks and the benefits will usually prevail if the indication is well based. The possibility of performing the operation using a combination of regional and general anaesthesia should also be considered. Indeed, this often provides the best anaesthesia for the patient. Only in exceptional cases should a patient be obliged to remain awake, if they have strong objections.

Premedication

This will depend upon the individual patient, whether or not he or she will remain conscious, and on the anaesthetist's preference. No premedicant drugs are contraindicated in regional anaesthesia.

Management during anaesthesia and surgery

During the preparation for, and the performance of, the local/regional anaesthesia, the way in which the patient is treated is of great importance. An accurate explanation of what is to happen step by step, will get the patient's confidence. If a concomitant general anaesthetic is planned, there is a temptation to put the patient "to sleep" before performing the local technique. This may indeed be desirable, e.g. in a child, but many techniques are better done with the patient conscious so as to assess such things as paraesthesia or accidental intravenous injection, before any general anaesthesia is given.

In all but the most trivial procedures, no local anaesthetic drug should be injected unless all the necessary apparatus (including that needed for monitoring) and drugs which may be required for resuscitation are at hand. In general these will be identical to those required for other types of anaesthesia.

Intravenous access is particularly important and should be ensured by an indwelling needle or IV infusion before the regional technique is performed.

The injection of local anaesthetic drug is of course the **start** and not the **end** of the anaesthesia. Once the block has been performed, the management will depend upon whether or not the patient is to remain awake or be rendered unconscious with a light general anaesthetic.

Conscious patients

Conscious patients will require special management which should include:

1. Delaying the operation, and its preparation, until the local anaesthetic has produced its full effect. Impatience in this respect is one of the commonest reasons for failure of regional anaesthesia.

2. Ensuring that **all** members of the surgical team are aware that the patient is conscious. Loud noises and injudicious conversation can greatly alarm patients who are usually quite unused to the operation room environment. Nurses, doctors and attendants should be calm, solicitous and considerate towards the patient.

3. The patient should be made comfortable on the operating table.

4. The patient should be reassured that the anaesthetist is always immediately available and able to deal with any problems.

5. If there is a complaint of pain or discomfort, the anaesthetist should explain the reason and treat it as indicated. It is never a good idea to tell the patient beforehand that he/she "will feel nothing". This is frequently untrue and the patient will lose confidence. Most patients will tolerate some discomfort if it is short-lived, e.g. during delivery of the baby's head at Caesarean section. If there is a deficiency in the effectiveness of the block, then an analgesic drug, preferably an opioid, should be given intravenously, e.g. morphine 10 mg, diamorphine 5 mg, pethidine 100 mg or fentanyl 100 μg. Do not treat pain initially with a sedative or tranquillising drug. These have no analgesic properties and frequently cause the patient to become irrational and uncooperative. The sedative properties of opioids are usually sufficient once they have controlled the pain.

6. If, in the absence of pain, the patient becomes frightened or hysterical, a tranquilliser such as diazepam 5-10 mg given slowly IV may become necessary. Remember that irrational and hysterical behaviour may be evidence of generalised toxicity to the local anaesthetic drug.

7. It may be decided before operation to give the patient moderate or deep sedation. Benzodiazepines are the most popular drugs for this purpose. They should be given in small IV increments, e.g. diazepam 1 mg every 30 s, until the desired level of sedation is reached. Intravenous chlormethiazole (0.8% as an infusion) is also very useful as the depth of sedation can be easily and quickly modified by adjustment of the infusion rate. Unlike when benzodiazepines are used, recovery to full lucidity will occur within minutes of stopping the infusion.

8. The patient's blood pressure should be carefully monitored, particularly with spinal or epidural block. Conscious patients tolerate decreases in their arterial pressure badly. Even a modest degree of hypotension may trigger a vasovagal attack with bradycardia (or even transient cardiac arrest), extreme hypotension, unconsciousness, nausea and vomiting.

9. Postoperatively patients with epidural or spinal blocks should be under medical and nursing observation until the local anaesthesia has worn off.

Concomitant general anaesthesia

General anaesthesia used alone has to meet a triad of requirements, namely, unconsciousness, analgesia and relaxation. The last two are usually achieved with specific drugs, i.e. opioids and muscle relaxants. As regional anaesthesia can provide analgesia (which is much superior in quality to that of opioids) and relaxation (confined to the operative area and not involving the muscles of respiration), the addition of a light general anaesthetic to a regional technique is quite logical. The following advantages accrue:

1. A patient's preference to be unconscious can be met. If the local anaesthesia is not adequate for any reason, the patient will be unaware of it though it will be obvious to the anaesthetist, who can deal with it appropriately.

2. Deep anaesthesia is not required and recovery of consciousness is rapid. On the other hand most of the agents used for sedation of a conscious patient are only slowly metabolised and complete recovery may be delayed for many hours.

3. Time is saved because preparations for the operation, e.g. positioning, cleaning the skin and catheterisation, can be made **before** the local anaesthetic is fully effective.

4. Spontaneous respiration is maintained and there is no requirement for paralysis and artificial ventilation.

5. Most patients will awaken in a pain-free state.

6. The stress on the operating team of having a conscious patient is removed.

7. Sudden hypotension as seen with vaso-vagal attacks does not occur in anaesthetised patients.

8. Hypotension is well tolerated and can indeed be used where indicated to reduce operative bleeding.

The general anaesthesia should be of the simplest type with an IV agent for induction followed by a weak concentration of an inhalational agent. Endotracheal intubation is seldom required provided the airway is kept quite clear. If preferred, a total intravenous anaesthetic can be given.

Monitoring during local/ regional anaesthesia

Like all patients being anaesthetised, those receiving local anaesthetics should be under continuous observation. The following are considered the minimal requirements:

Pulse
A palpable pulse gives information on the pulse rate and the presence of arrhythmias and is an indication of arterial pressure and cardiac output, particularly if these change rapidly.

ECG
This accurately calculates heart rate, defines an arrhythmia and may show evidence of myocardial ischaemia. A tachycardia seen during or soon after the injection of local anaesthetic may be due to accidental IV injection if epinephrine has

been added to the solution. A slow heart rate (55-65 beats/min) may occur when a high sympathetic block occurs and cardiac accelerator nerves are affected. Marked bradycardia (less than 55 beats/min) should warn of a vaso-vagal attack, if the patient is conscious.

Arterial pressure

Non-invasive monitoring of blood pressure is quite adequate in most cases. An automatic machine has many advantages, particularly if the anaesthetist is working alone.

Respiration

Paralysis of the respiratory muscles, particularly the intercostals, may occur with high spinal or epidural block. This will be suggested by dyspnoea and indrawing of the intercostal muscles during inspiration. If a general anaesthetic is being given then the airway and the volume of gas being shifted during respiration should be checked continuously. Irregularity of breathing and breath holding may indicate inadequacy of analgesia and/or too light anaesthesia.

Blood loss

Patients with widespread sympathetic block are less tolerant of blood loss and appropriate fluid replacement must be timely.

More elaborate invasive monitoring including arterial, central venous pulmonary artery and wedge pressure, may be required in special circumstances.

Local anaesthetic drugs

All local anaesthetic drugs have a common molecular structure and a similar mode of action. There are many drugs available and they differ to a greater or lesser extent in regard to:

1. Potency
2. Onset time or latency
3. Duration of effect
4. Toxicity

Thus the choice of drug will be mainly influenced by the individual patient's requirements.

Unlike most other drugs, local anaesthetics are applied or injected at their site of action, i.e. close to the nerves to be blocked. As a result their **local** concentration is several orders of magnitude greater than their **plasma** concentration after absorption. This accounts not only for their relative safety if they are properly injected in the correct dose, but also for their potential danger if they are injected IV by accident, or an overdose is given.

Chemical structure

All commonly used local anaesthetics have a three-part structure:

Aromatic ring - Intermediate chain - Amino group.

As the intermediate chain contains either an ester or an amide linkage, they may conveniently be divided into esters and amides.

Ester linkage $-COO-$

An ester linkage is relatively unstable and ester local anaesthetics are broken down by hydrolysis both in solution and, following injection, in the plasma by pseudocholinesterase. Thus solutions have a relatively short shelf-life and are difficult to sterilise as heat cannot be used. Because they are broken down in the plasma, they can be relatively non-toxic if this process is rapid, as with procaine and chloroprocaine, but in such cases their duration of effect is also brief.

Amide linkage $-NHCO-$

An amide linkage is much more stable than an ester, and the drugs in solution withstand heat sterilisation and changes in pH (which may be necessary when adding epinephrine). Likewise they are not broken down in plasma and must be metabolised by the liver, as little or no drug is excreted unchanged.

Table 1
Physicochemical Properties of Local Anaesthetics

Agent	Aromatic Lipophillic	Intermediate Chain	Amine Hydrophillic	Molecular Weight (base)	pKa (25°C)	Partition Coefficient	% Protein Binding
Esters							
Procaine	$H-N-\bigcirc-$	$COOCH_2CH_2$	$-N(C_2H_5)_2$	236	8.9	0.02	5.8
Tetracaine	$H_9C_4N-\bigcirc-$	$COOCH_2CH_2$	$-N(CH_3)_2$	264	8.6	4.1	75.6
Chloroprocaine	$H-N-\bigcirc-$ (Cl)	$COOCH_2CH_2$	$-N(C_2H_5)_2$	271	8.7	0.14	—
Amides							
Prilocaine	(CH₃ aromatic)	$NHCOCH(CH_3)$	$-N(H)(C_3H_7)$	220	7.7	0.9	55 approx.
Lidocaine	(2,6-dimethyl aromatic)	$NHCOCH_2$	$-N(C_2H_5)_2$	234	7.7	2.9	64.3
Mepivacaine	(2,6-dimethyl aromatic)	$NHCO$	N-methyl piperidine	246	7.6	0.8	77.5
Bupivacaine	(2,6-dimethyl aromatic)	$NHCO$	N-butyl (C_4H_9) piperidine	288	8.1	27.5	95.6
Etidocaine	(2,6-dimethyl aromatic)	$NHCOCH(C_2H_5)$	$-N(C_2H_5)(C_3H_7)$	276	7.7	141	94

Physicochemical properties

Local anaesthetics vary in regard to their lipid/water solubility ratio, their pKa and the degree to which they bind to protein (Table 1).

Lipid solubility is the main determinant of potency: the higher the lipid/water partition coefficient, the more potent the drug is likely to be.

Protein binding determines the duration of effect, presumably because highly bound drugs stay in the lipoprotein of nerve membranes longer.

The pKa of a compound determines how much is ionised and how much is unionised when injected into the body. Thus the higher the pKa, the less of the unionised base form is present. As only unionised drug can penetrate nerve membranes, the pKa will affect the speed of onset of the drugs: the lower the pKa, the faster the onset (Table 2).

Table 2..

Relationship of pKa to percent bas form and time for 50 conduction block in isolated nerve

Agent	pKa	% Base at pH 7.4	Onset (min)
Prilocaine	7.7	35	2-4
Lidocaine	7.7	35	2-4
Etidocaine	7.7	35	2-4
Bupivacaine	8.1	20	5-8
Tetracaine	8.6	5	10-15
Procaine	8.9	2	14-18

Mode of action

Local anaesthetics cause a reversible block to the conduction of impulses along nerve fibres. A propagated nerve impulse involves a wave of depolarisation, followed by repolarisation, passing along the nerve fibre. In the resting mode, nerve fibres are polarised, with higher concentrations of sodium ions outside than inside the cell, and the reverse for potassium ions (Fig. 1).

Depolarisation is caused by a flow of sodium ions through sodium channels in the nerve membrane, from the the outside to the inside of the nerve fibres (Fig. 2).

Fig. 1.

Fig. 2.

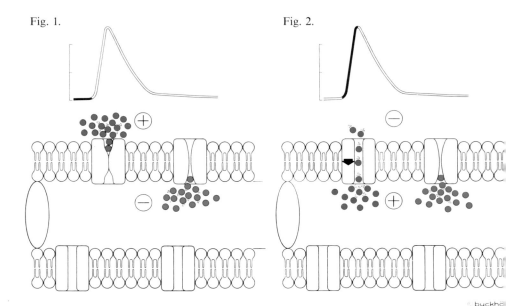

buckhö

Repolarisation involves the flow, in the reverse direction, of potassium ions (Fig. 3).

The resultant slight imbalance of ions (too much Na inside and too much K outside) is corrected after repolarisation by ionic pumps (Fig. 4).

The electrical spike caused by depolarisation triggers the adjacent membrane, such that the sodium channels in that section of the fibre open in their turn, allowing the inward flow of sodium ions and depolarisation. Thus each depolarisation/repolarisation that occurs triggers a similar process in the adjacent membrane and this passes along the nerve from one end to the other.

Fig. 3.

Fig. 4.

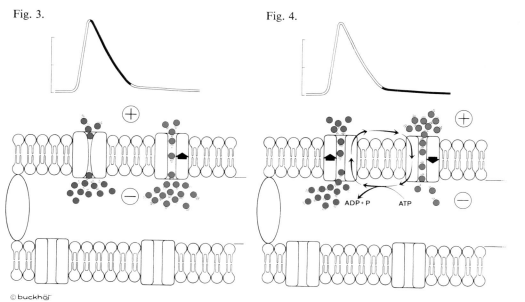

© buckhöj

Local anaesthetics cause changes in the nerve membrane which prevent depolarisation and thus block nerve propagation, a process termed "stabilising the membrane". They achieve this by preventing the sodium channels opening, thus maintaining the fully polarised state (Fig. 5).

Most local anaesthetics are relatively insoluble in water and are prepared as the soluble hydrochloride salt. When this is injected, it ionises into positively charged anions of the local anaesthetic and negative charged chloride ions, i.e.

$$LA\ HCl \longrightarrow LAH^+ + Cl^-$$

As the anionic form must also dissociate at the body pH, the following reaction occurs:

$$LAH^+ \rightleftharpoons LA + H^+$$

Anion   Base

Thus after injection of the hydrochloride salt, both the charged anionic form and the uncharged basic form of the compound rapidly appear. The proportion of charged/uncharged forms depends upon the pKa of the drug. Local anaesthetics have pKa's above 7.4 and the greater the pKa, the greater the amount of the uncharged form that is present.

Only the lipid soluble uncharged form of the drug can penetrate the epineurium and the nerve membrane. The membrane made up of an lipid bilayer and protein molecules that contain the sodium channels (Fig. 6). The axoplasm, however, is a watery milieu and on reaching it after passage through the membrane, the uncharged base must again dissociate and form a mixture of both the charged and uncharged forms. The charged anionic form of the local anaesthetic then gains access to the sodium channels ring and renders them incapable of allowing sodium ions to pass through the membrane. Nerve impulses cannot then be propagated and nerve block ensues. As the block develops depolarisation is first slowed, and then finally prevented.

Fig. 5.

Fig. 6.

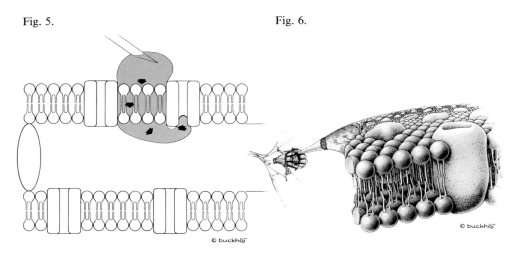

© buckhöj

© buckhöj

Other modes of action

Benzocaine (sodium para-aminobenzoate) does not ionise at body pH and thus only exists in the base form. It can enter the membrane but will not reach the axoplasm. It is thought to act by membrane expansion which will physically occlude the sodium channels, a mechanism similar to that of general anaesthetics on the brain.

Conversely, the biotoxins e.g. tetradotoxin and saxitoxin, which are highly potent local anaesthetics, only exist in the charged ionised form and cannot enter the membrane. To block nerve conduction they must attach themselves to the outer part of the sodium channels. This process is shown in Fig. 7.

Choice of local anaesthetic drug

In choosing a local anaesthetic drug and the appropriate concentration, the factors to be borne in mind are:

Specific nerves to be blocked
Small nerves are in general much easier to block than large ones. Thus nerve endings and small cutaneous nerves are easily and quickly blocked by low concentrations of drugs given by infiltration. Large nerves with thick perineurium are much more difficult and require high concentrations of drug. However, the large spinal nerves within the subarachnoid space have no perineurium and are easily blocked.

It is generally held that motor fibres are the most difficult to block, followed by somatic sensory and autonomic fibres in descending order. However, there is evidence that the small C fibres, can be relatively resistant to local anaesthetics.

Onset time or latency
A rapid onset may be required, e.g. for an urgent operation or to relieve acute pain. In such cases an agent with a rapid onset can be used or an alternative procedure may be performed e.g. a spinal block instead of an epidural block.

Epinephrine can decrease latency (vide infra).

Required duration of effect
The duration of local anaesthetics may vary from 30 min to 180 min or longer. Moreover duration is related to the dosage, increasing which gives a longer duration. Clearly the duration should outlast the operation. Thereafter the optimal duration will depend upon the desirability of postoperative analgesia and the need to regain full function.

The duration can be increased by adding epinephrine to the local anaesthetic (vide infra). When very prolonged anaesthesia is required, an indwelling plastic catheter may be used, and repeat injections of local anaesthetic made as required.

For permanent nerve blockade, neurolytic agents such as phenol or alcohol are employed.

Fig. 7.

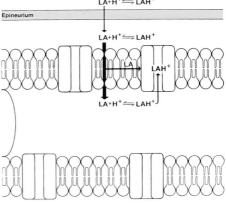

© buckhöj

21

Drug properties

Lidocaine HCl

(Carbonated salt also available in some countries).

Short onset, medium duration drug. 0.5-2% for injection, 4-10% for topical application. Used for all forms of regional anaesthesia. Also used for treatment of ventricular arrhythmias.

Prilocaine HCl

Short onset, medium duration drug. Significantly less toxic than lidocaine. Causes methaemoglobinaemia in doses over 600 mg; thus not suitable for continuous analgesia. 0.5-2% for injection. Specially indicated for high doses techniques (e.g. plexus blockade) and for IV regional anaesthesia (Bier's block).

Mepivacaine HCl

Short onset, medium duration drug. Less toxic than lidocaine. 0.5-2% for injection.

Bupivacaine HCl

(Carbonated salt also available in some countries).

Long onset, long duration. 0.125-0.75% for injection (0.75% has short onset). Causes less motor block than most other local anaesthetics at concentrations of 0.5% or less; hence valuable for prolonged analgesia. More cardiotoxic than equipotent concentrations of lidocaine.

Chloroprocaine HCl

Short onset, short acting drug. Low toxicity due to rapid hydrolysis in plasma. 1-3% for injection. Neuropathy has been described, but this was probably due to added metabisulphite and the formulation has now been changed. 3% gives rapid onset for Caesarean sections done with epidural block.

Procaine HCl

Slow onset, short duration drug. Now seldom used. 1-2% for injection. Useful for short duration spinal anaesthesia.

Tetracaine HCl

Slow onset, long duration drug. Main use is in spinal anaesthesia and for topical application. Rather toxic if used for nerve blocks.

Dosage of local anaesthetic drugs

There are few areas in anaesthesia where dosage recommendations are more confused than in regional anaesthesia. This is in large part due to the insistence of the various national pharmacopoeias and regulatory authorities on laying down a "maximum recommended dose" for local anaesthetic drugs. Such a restriction does not apply to other classes of drug. The avoidance of toxicity is of course very important, but toxicity seldom arises if the local anaesthetic is injected correctly. The commonest cause of toxicity is accidental IV injection and a "maximum recommended dose" of any local anaesthetic given as a fast bolus injection will still cause overt toxicity with convulsions.

The problem is compounded by the fact that the peak plasma concentration following absorption from a correctly placed injection depends primarily on the site of injection. Thus an intercostal block gives over 3 times the peak concentration that follows a subcutaneous injection in an abdominal field block. Clearly then the "maximum recommended dose" should be adjusted for each site of injection.

There is a particular difficulty with lidocaine, the most widely used local anaesthetic. Since its introduction over 30 years ago it has been stated that the maximum recommended dose is 200 mg of plain solution and 500 mg of an epinephrine containing solution. Nothing could be more illogical, the former dose being far too small and the latter making the

incorrect assumption that epinephrine allows a 150% increase in dosage. For these reasons the author has doubled the recommended dose for plain solutions of lidocaine, but it should be understood that this is a personal view, not accepted at the present time by the regulatory authorities. Many, and probably most, experts in the field, however, would agree that 400 mg of plain lidocaine will not cause overt toxicity unless it is given accidentally into a blood vessel.

The relative potencies of the common local anaesthetic drugs are given in Table 3.

Table 3.
Comparative potencies of local anaesthestics (%)

Lidocaine	0.5	1	1.5	2	
Mepivacaine	0.5	1	1.5	2	
Prilocaine	0.5	1	1.5	2	
Bupivacaine	0.125	0.25	0.375	0.5	0.75
Etidocaine	0.25	0.5	0.75	1	1.5
Chloroprocaine	0.5	1	1.5	2	3
Procaine	1	2			

The doses recommended for epidural block (Table 4) (which requires the highest concentration of local anaesthetics), and the doses likely to cause convulsions if given IV by fast bolus injection in adults, are given in Table 4. The onset times and durations are also included.

Table 4. Maximum epidural dose, toxicity, speed of onset and duration of effect of the common local anaesthetics

Drug	Maximum dose epidurally	Toxic dose if IV	Onset to surgical analgesia (min)	Duration (min)
Lidocaine 2%	20 ml (400 mg)	12.5 ml (250 mg)	10-20	90-120
Lidocaine 2% with epinephrine	25 ml (500 mg)	12.5 ml (250 mg)	7-15	120-180
Prilocaine 2%	25 ml (500 mg)	17.5 ml (350 mg)	10-20	90-120
Prilocaine 2% with epinephrine	30 ml (600 mg)	17.5 ml (350 mg)	7-15	120-180
Mepivacaine 2%	25 ml (400 mg)	17.5 ml (350 mg)	10-20	90-120
Mepivacaine 2% with epinephrine	30 ml (600 mg)	17.5 ml (350 mg)	7-15	120-180
Bupivacaine 0.5%	20 ml (100 mg)	16.0 ml (80 mg)	20-40	180-240
Bupivacaine 0.5% with epinephrine	25 ml (125 mg)	16.0 ml (80 mg)	15-30	200-300
Bupivacaine 0.75%	20 ml (150 mg)	11.0 ml (80 mg)	15-30	250-400
Bupivacaine 0.75% with epinephrine	25 ml (182.5 mg)	11.0 ml (80 mg)	10-20	250-450
Etidocaine 1.5%	20 ml (300 mg)	12.0 ml (180 mg)	10-20	200-300
Etidocaine 1.5% with epinephrine	25 ml (375 mg)	12.0 ml (180 mg)	7-15	250-420
Chloroprocaine 3%	20 ml (600 mg)	15.0 ml (450 mg)	10-20	45-60
Chloroprocaine 3% with epinephrine	25 ml (750 mg)	15.0 ml (450 mg)	7-15	60-80

Toxicity of local anaesthetic drugs

There is not a great difference in toxicity between equipotent doses of most local anaesthetics but it is best to use one of low toxicity when large doses are required (e.g. for brachial plexus block) or when IV regional anaesthesia is used.

Systemic toxicity of local anaesthetic drugs

The effect of local anaesthetic drugs on sodium channels in nerve membranes ensures that if toxic effects do occure they will be in organs with excitable membranes, particularly the brain and the myocardium. All those who use potentially toxic doses of local anaesthetics should be aware of the possibility of toxic reactions and know how to recognise and treat them.

The systemic toxicity of local anaesthetic drugs depends upon:

1. Dose

2. Site of injection
Vascular sites lead to rapid absorption. Thus intercostal injection gives much higher plasma concentrations than subcutaneous injection. Accidental IV injection is the commonest cause of toxicity.

3. Drug used
The drugs of lowest toxicity are prilocaine, mepivacaine, chloroprocaine and procaine.

4. Speed of injection
This is only of importance if the drug is given IV, when fast injections will achieve much higher plasma concentrations than slow injections. Injecting small aliquots over several minutes prolongs the administration and will reduce toxicity when high dosage is required, e.g. in epidural, intercostal or major plexus blocks.

5. Addition of epinephrine
This causes local vasoconstriction and slows absorption. It is more effective at subcutaneous sites than elsewhere but a reduction in the peak concentration of between 20% and 50% may be anticipated with most local anaesthetics.

Signs and symptoms of toxicity

Local anaesthetics have their major toxic effects in the brain and myocardium. The brain is more susceptible than the heart and all the early signs and symptoms are related to CNS toxicity, serious myocardial dysfunction only being seen with excessive plasma concentrations.

Central nervous system toxicity

Central nervous system toxicity involves a spectrum of signs and symptoms from mild to serious. In increasing order of severity, the following may occur:

1. Numbness of the mouth and tongue
2. Lightheadedness
3. Tinnitus
4. Visual disturbance
5. Irrational behaviour and speech
6. Muscle twitching
7. Unconsciousness
8. Generalised convulsions
9. Coma
10. Apnoea

CNS toxicity will be enhanced by acidosis and hypoxia, both of which can occur very rapidly if convulsions appear, when breathing may stop and the excessive muscular activity consumes oxygen stores.

Cardiovascular toxicity

Cardiovascular toxicity is due to slowing of conduction in the myocardium, myocardial depression and peripheral vasodilatation. It is usually only seen clinically after 2-4 times the convulsant dose has been injected. Hypotension, bradycardia and eventually cardiac standstill may occur. An exception to this is with bupivacaine, which can affect conduction within the myocardium at relatively low plasma concentrations. As a result sudden ventricular fibrillation has been seen with this drug after rapid IV injection.

Prevention of toxicity

Local anaesthetic toxicity can be avoided in most cases by a few simple rules:

1. Always use the recommended dose.

2. Aspirate through the needle or catheter before injecting the local anaesthetic.

3. Use a test dose containing epinephrine when appropriate. If the needle or catheter is within a vein, the test dose will produce an acute increase in heart rate 30-45 s after the injection. The duration of the tachycardia is brief and a continous ECG is recommended.

4. If a large quantity of drug is required or if the drug is given IV on purpose (e.g. for IV regional anaesthesia) use a drug of low toxicity, and divide the dose into smaller aliquots, spreading the time taken for the total injection.

5. Always inject slowly (not faster than 10 ml/min) and maintain verbal contact with the patient, who can report minor symptoms before the entire intended dose is given. Beware of the patient who starts to speak and act irrationally. It is probably due to CNS toxicity but may be mistaken for hysteria.

Treatment of toxicity

Provided the diagnosis is borne in mind, toxicity may be recognised early and effective treatment given without delay. All necessary equipment and drugs should be available **before** injecting local anaesthetic. The two cardinal rules are:

1. Give oxygen, if necessary by artificial respiration using a bag and mask.

2. Stop the convulsions if they continue for more than 15-20 s. To do this an anticonvulsant must be given IV, e.g. thiopental 100-150 mg or diazepam 5-20 mg. The former is usually more readily available and is quicker acting. Some authorities prefer to give succinylcholine 50-100 mg, which will quickly stop the convulsions but will require intubation and artificial ventilation until the effects have worn off.

Toxicity can disappear as quickly as it appears and a decision must then be made whether to postpone surgery, repeat the nerve block, use a different technique (e.g. give a spinal instead of an epidural block) or change to general anaesthesia.

If hypotension and signs of myocardial depression occur, a vasopressor with both α- and β-adrenergic activity should be given, e.g. ephedrine 15-30 mg IV. Cardiac standstill must be treated by energetic cardiopulmonary resuscitation including IV or intracardiac epinephrine 1 mg and atropine 0.6 mg. Ventricular fibrillation should be treated by high energy DC conversion plus bretylium 80 mg as an anti-arrhythmic.

Sensitivity to local anaesthetic drugs

Sensitivity or allergy is excessively rare in the case of amide local anaesthetics but is occasionally seen with esters. Other constituents within an ampoule or vial of local anaesthetic e.g. methylparaben, may be responsible for some reactions.

Patients may claim to be sensitive, usually as a result of an unpleasant experience in the course of dental treatment. Most likely the patient fainted or felt faint and this was wrongly labelled as sensitivity.

If there is any doubt the patient should be given a skin test which, if negative, may be followed by a challenge using a small subcutaneous dose. This should only be done in a properly equipped area so that if allergy occurs it can be promptly treated.

Other drugs used in regional anaesthesia

Epinephrine

This may be added to local anaesthetic solutions to increase their effectiveness and to reduce toxicity. It causes a local vasoconstriction and delays absorption from the site of injection. Thus the local anaesthetic is in contact with the target nerves for a longer time. As a result the latency is reduced, the block is more effective and the duration is increased. Slowing the absorption also decreases the peak plasma concentration.

Epinephrine works better at some locations than others, being most effective at subcutaneous sites.

The optimal concentration is 1:200.000, i.e. 5 μg/ml. Local anaesthetics containing epinephrine are available commercially. Alternatively the epinephrine may be added immediately before use, 0.1 ml of 1:1.000 (i.e. 100 μg) being added to 20 ml of local anaesthetic.

It is unwise to inject epinephrine near terminal arteries, e.g. digital arteries, for fear of causing tissue necrosis and gangrene.

Other local vasoconstrictors

Although many agents have been tried, none appears to have any advantage over epinephrine. The only drug which has achieved popularity is felypressin (Octapressin), which is added to prilocaine for dental use.

Parenteral vasopressors

These drugs are used to prevent or correct hypotension resulting from sympathetic blockade in spinal or epidural anaesthesia.

The commonest of these are:

Ephedrine

This is sympathomimetic with both α- and β-receptor activity. Given IV in a dose of 10-15 mg it rapidly (60-90 s) raises arterial pressure, and this effect lasts for 15-30 min. Occasionally larger doses may be required. Given IM it takes 10-15 min to work and it lasts up to 1 h. It is logical, therefore, for rapid effect and long duration, to give enough drug IV to restore the pressure, and the same dose IM. The IM route can also be used prophylactically to prevent decreases in arterial pressure, e.g. just after injecting the local anaesthetic for spinal or epidural anaesthesia.

Phenylephrine

Phenylephrine is a pure α-receptor agonist, and must be given by IV infusion. 10-20 mg is diluted in 500 ml of saline or dextrose and infused, the dose being titrated to the desired effect.

Methoxamine

Methoxamine (Vasoxine) is an α-receptor agonist and a β-blocker. It raises pressure but slows the heart rate with a consequent decrease in cardiac output. This unusual combination of effects makes it theoretically the best drug to use in patients with coronary insufficiency because it should increase coronary flow (by increasing afterload) and decrease myocardial work (by decreasing cardiac output). Both the IM and IV routes can be used and the dosage is 10-30 mg.

Dihydroergotamine

Dihydroergotamine has been used both to treat and to prevent hypotension. It differs from sympathomimetics in that its main effect is vasoconstriction on the venous side of the circulation, causing a decrease in venous capacitance and an increase in venous return. It also causes a mild degree of arteriolar vasoconstriction. Arterial pressure returns towards normal without overshoot or tachycardia. The dose is 0.5-1 mg and it can be used IV or IM. It has been found to decrease liver blood flow.

Complications of regional anaesthesia

The complications of regional anaesthesia may be divided into immediate, intermediate and late.

Immediate complications

Toxic reactions

See p. 25.

Hypotension

Hypotension is usually associated with widespread sympathetic blockade and therefore with spinal or epidural block. However, even high blocks involving most of the sympathetic outflow are not associated with severe hypotension in the majority of patients, only about 25% suffering a decrease in systolic pressure greater than 30 mmHg. Additional factors precipitating severe hypotension are:

1. Hypovolaemia
2. Fainting due to vaso-vagal attack
3. Inferior vena caval occlusion in late pregnancy or in the presence of large abdominal tumour.

Hypotension may be prevented by giving a fluid load (e.g., 1 litre of Hartmann's solution) just before performing the block, or by giving a vasopressor. Caval occlusion may be avoided by turning the patient into a semilateral position, or using uterine displacement.

As hypotension only occurs in a minority of patients, some authorities prefer to await its development, and treat it as required, using an IV vasopressor (see p. 28).

Respiratory paralysis

Respiratory paralysis can occur with the inadvertent injection of a large quantity of local anaesthetic into the subarachnoid or subdural space instead of the epidural space. Very occasionally it can occur with an unduly high epidural or spinal block. The patient will complain of dyspnoea and the intercostal muscles will be indrawn during inspiration. If the phrenic nerve is paralysed (C3, 4, 5), respiration will cease. Treatment is by artificial respiration until the paralysis wears off.

Patients who faint may also complain of dyspnoea, which is due to air hunger consequent on the very low cardiac output. Extreme bradycardia due to vagal overactivity, in the presence of good respiratory movement, will suggest this diagnosis.

Pain on injection

Acute pain referred to the distribution of the nerve being blocked is a serious event as it indicates an intraneural injection. The injection should be stopped immediately as nerve damage can occur. This shooting type pain should not be confused with the dull aching pain which can occur when large volumes are injected into a confined space, e.g. with brachial plexus block.

Intermediate complications

Motor paralysis

If it occurs within the operative area, muscle paralysis is usually beneficial. However, in the case of epidural and spinal anaesthesia, paralysis of the lower limbs may be a problem as some patients are disturbed by it, especially if the regional block is being used for prolonged pain relief, e.g. in labour or postoperatively. Reassurance of the patient is essential and the use of lower concentrations of drug at subsequent injections will usually allow more active movement of the lower limbs.

Paralysis of the respiratory muscles is mentioned above.

Urinary retention

The parasympathetic motor nerves to the bladder arise from the spinal segments S2, 3 and 4. The sympathetic sensory nerves enter the spinal cord via T11-L2. Thus spinal and epidural blocks at these levels can cause urinary retention and require bladder catheterisation. As patients may not be aware of their distending bladder, they must be observed both in regard to urinary output and a palpable bladder. Catheterisation is often condemned because of the possibility of urinary infection and bacteraemia. Repeated aseptic catheterisation is thought to carry less risk of infection than continuous drainage, but the great majority of patients will suffer little or no harm from catheterisation. Many pelvic and perineal operations require catheterisation regardless of the anaesthesia. Prophylactic antibiotics will prevent infection becoming establisted.

Late complications

Neurological damage

Neurological damage which may be long-lasting or even permanent is the most feared complication of regional anaesthesia. There are several causes for such damage occurring (Table 5).

Should a neurological complication occur, or be suspected, an expert neurological opinion should be urgently sought. If a space-occupying lesion is suspected, an emergency laminectomy may be necessary. Otherwise a careful history and examination will elucidate the diagnosis and determine the presence and extent of any pre-existing disease.

The main causes of neurological problems are:

Nerve trauma

Apart from the damage to nerve fibres caused by a needle or catheter entering a nerve, the injection of local anaesthetic directly into a nerve can physically disrupt the fibres and may lead to neuropathy.

Anterior spinal artery syndrome

This causes paraplegia and is due to occlusion or inadequate flow in the artery of Adamkiewicz, which supplies the lower third of the spinal cord. The main cause of inadequate flow is hypotension in the presence of local arteriosclerosis.

Adhesive arachnoiditis

This may follow the injection of an irritant or infected solution into the epidural or subarachnoid space.

A space-occupying lesion

A space-occupying lesion in the spinal canal, e.g. haematoma or abscess, can cause paraplegia, and may or may not be associated with the injection of local anaesthetic.

Table 5
Summary of various types of neurological damage following epidural blockade

Pathology	Cause	Onset	Clinical features	Outcome
Spinal nerve neuropathy	Trauma (needle, catheter, injection)	0-2 days	Pain during insertion of needle or catheter. Pain on injection. Paraesthesia, pain and numbness over distribution of spinal nerve.	Recovery 1-12 weeks
Anterior spinal artery sydrome	Arteriosclerosis Hypotension	Immediate	Postoperative painless paraplegia.	Painless paraplegia.
Adhesive arachnoiditis	Irritant injectate	0-7 days	Pain on injection. Variable degree of neurological deficit. Often progressive with pain and paraplegia.	May progress to severe disability with pain and paralysis.
Space -occupying lesion (haematoma or abscess)	Hypocoagulation Bacteraemia	0-2 days	Severe backache postoperatively with progressive paraplegia.	Requires immediate surgery, otherwise paraplegia.

Pneumothorax

Pneumothorax is a complication of intercostal nerve block and supraclavicular brachial plexus block. It should be kept in mind after performing these blocks. A chest X-ray will quickly make the diagnosis. Treatment will depend upon the amount of air in the pleural cavity and the adequacy of respiratory function.

Headache

Headache can follow the piercing of the dura mater in the course of spinal anaesthesia or when it is punctured accidentally during attempted epidural block. The headache is due to low cerebrospinal fluid pressure. Treatment is given on p. 79.

Drug nomenclature

Throughout this book we have used the World Health Organisation's International Non-proprietary Name (INN) convention. The alternative names of the various drugs, whether proprietary or generic, are given in Table 6.

Table 6. Drug nomenclature

INN	Other names

Local anaesthetics

Bupivacaine	Marcaine, Sensorcaine, Carbostesin
Chloroprocaine	2-Chlorprocaine, Nesacaine
Eitdocaine	Duranest
Lidocaine	Lignocaine, Xylocaine
Mepivacaine	Carbocaine
Prilocaine	Citanest
Procaine	Novocaine
Tetracaine	Amethocaine, Anethaine, Pontocaine, Pantocaine

Vasopressors & Sympathomimetics

Epinephrine	Adrenaline
Ephedrine	-
Methoxamine	Vasoxine, Vasoxyl
Norepinephrine	Noradrenaline, Levophed
Phenylephrine	Neosynephrine

Opioids

Fentanyl	Sublimaze
Hydromorphone	Dilaudid
Methadone	Amidone, Phenodone, Physeptone, Dolophine
Morphine	-
Naloxone	Narcan
Pethidine	Meperidine, Demerol, Dolantin

Other drugs

Chlormethiazole	Heminevrine, Hemineurine
Diazepam	Valium
Midazolam	Hypnovel
Oxytocin	Syntocinon, Syntometrine, Uteracon
Temazepam	Normison, Euhypros
Thiopental	Pentothal, Thiopentone

Aids to regional anaesthesia

Because it is necessary with many techniques of regional anaesthesia to inject the local anaesthetic solution as close as possible to the appropriate nerves, several methods are available to help the anaesthetist determine the anatomy accurately.

Elicitation of paraesthesia

If a sensory nerve is touched by a hypodermic needle a paraesthesia in the distribution of the nerve will occur. While this is used to identify the nerve for many blocks it is important not to damage the nerve. Thus long bevelled and very sharp needles are to be avoided. Patient cooperation is of course essential.

Nerve stimulator

By passing small electric pulses down the injection needle, the proximity of the needle point to the nerve can be determined, as twitching in the muscles supplied by the nerve begins as the needle approaches it. Provided excess current is not used, this is not painful for the patient. The position in which the twitch is maximal gives the nearest position to the nerve. Nerve stimulation can be used even in heavily sedated patients. The following points must be borne in mind:

1. The nerve stimulator must be able to deliver impulses of varying intensity from 0.2-5 mA at a frequency of 1 per second and a duration of 50-200 μs. Several machines are available commercially and those used for determining neuromuscular block are usually satisfactory. Approximate location to within 2 cm of the nerve is achieved using a current of 2-5 mA but this should be reduced to 0.2-0.5 mA when approaching close to the nerve. The current used will depend upon the duration of the stimulating impulse and it should therefore be adjustable and indicated on a dial or digital display.

2. While an ordinary needle can be used it is better to employ an insulated needle and it should be connected to the negative electrode. This ensures greater accuracy. The needle may be specially designed for the purpose but an IV needle and plastic cannula can easily be adapted to receive the electrical current. (Remember that IV needles are very sharp.)

3. Once muscle twitching in the nerve distribution at low current is obtained the injection of 1 ml of local anaesthetic (or any other solution) will immediately abolish the twitch, confirming close proximity between the needle tip and the nerve. The nerve stimulator can also be used to elicit paraesthesia when the nerve to be blocked does not contain motor fibres, e.g. the ophthalmic and maxillary divisions of the trigeminal nerve. It requires a higher current than that which produces muscular twitching.

Ultrasound

Some nerves have a close anatomical relationship to large arteries, identification of which is essential to success. In this people this seldom presents a problem but it can be quite difficult in muscular or fat patients. Excessive finger pressure used to feel the arterial pulsations can distort the position of the artery. Ultrasound will identify the correct position of the artery to within 1-2 mm without distortion and is particularly useful in brachial plexus block and femoral nerve block.

Immobile needle

With many nerve blocks it is essential that, having located the nerve, the needle is not moved during the injection. It is therefore not possible to hold the needle, connect the syringe and make the injection oneself. However, using a plastic extension tube to join the needle to the syringe, it is easy for the injection to be made by an assistant without the anaesthetist having to move either hand.

Radiological control

For some blocks where a neurolytic procedure is to be carried out, e.g. coeliac plexus block, it is essential to confirm the accurate placement of the neurolytic agent. This can be greatly simplified by the use of an image intensifier. The position of the needle tip can be checked, and when considered satisfactory, a small amount of radio-opaque dye is injected to eliminate misplacement. The main injection is only made when the correct position has been confirmed. Radio-opaque dye added to the neurolytic agent will also act as a useful check that the injection has been made in the correct location.

Figs. 9 and 10. Courtesy of Dr. G.L.M. Carmichael

Fig 9.

Fig. 10.

Fig. 8.

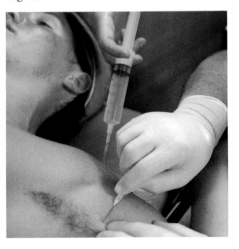

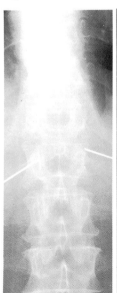

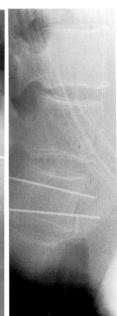

Brachial plexus block

Fig. 11.

1. First rib
2. Clavicle
3. Subclavian vein
4. Subclavian artery
5. Anterior scalene muscle
6. Middle scalene muscle
7. Transverse process of C6

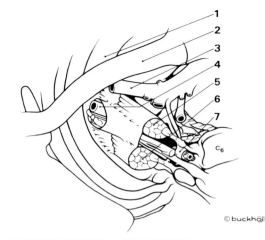

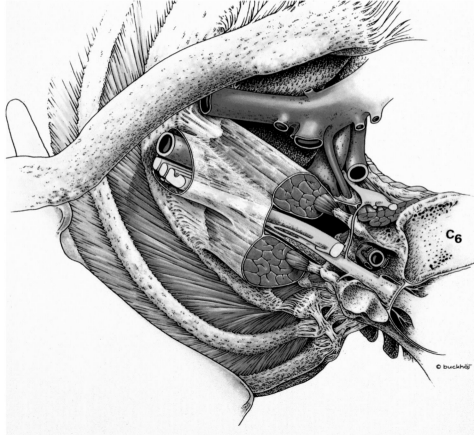

Anatomy

The brachial plexus is formed principally from the arterior primary rami of the C5, C6, C7, C8 and T1 spinal nerves. It runs from the vertebral column, passes between clavicle and first rib and enters the upper limb in the axilla before dividing into its four main terminal branches, the median, the radial, the ulnar and the musculo-cutaneous nerves. (Fig. 11.).

The plexus may be blocked with local anaesthetic at any point in its course from the neck to the axilla. The three commonest approaches are the interscalene, the supraclavicular and the axillary. Because the surrounding connective tissue forms a tube, the perivascular sheath, which contains the nerves and the main blood vessels of the upper limb, local anaesthetic can spread up and down inside this sheath regardless of the point of needle insertion. Theoretically an identical block will be obtained if sufficient anaesthetic solution is injected. However, this may require an excessive amount of drug. Given in smaller amounts, each of the three approaches gives a somewhat different distribution of anaesthesia. The choice between the three therefore depends upon the individual patient and the type of surgery to be undertaken.

Because large doses of local anaesthetic, often exceeding the maximum recommended dose may be required, it is advisable to use drugs of low toxicity such as prilocaine or mepivacaine.

Interscalene brachial plexus block
Anatomy

The brachial plexus in the neck runs between the anterior and middle scalene muscles. The perivascular sheath containing the plexus can be reached at the level of the 6th cervical vertebra, i.e. the same level as the cricoid cartilage (Fig. 12). This is some distance from either the subclavian artery or the dome of the pleura.

Patient position

Supine with upper limb at side. Head rotated a little away from the side to be blocked.

Landmarks

1. The groove between the anterior and middle scalene muscles. This is usually easily palpated behind the sternomastoid muscle, which is identified by asking the patient to raise his/her head. The muscle immediately behind the sternomastoid is

Fig. 12.

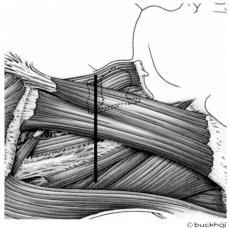

© buckhöj

the anterior scalene and by rolling the fingers backwards, the groove will be felt before reaching the middle scalene muscle.

2. Cricoid cartilage. This gives the level at which the needle should be inserted into the interscalene groove.

Needle insertion

A short needle (3-4 cm) may be used and is inserted perpendicular to the skin, i.e. medially but slightly downward and backward (Fig. 13). The index and middle finger of the non-dominant hand should be palpating the interscalene groove and preventing movement of the skin during needle insertion, which should be slightly closer to the middle than to the anterior scalene muscle. The needle is advanced **slowly** until a paraesthesia is elicited (Figs. 13 and 14), or a transverse spinous process is contacted.

The paraesthesia must be felt **below the shoulder,** as those felt above the clavicle may be due to contact with the supraclavicular nerve, which is outside the perivascular sheath. If bone, the transverse processes of the cervical vertebra, is contacted without paraesthesia it should be withdrawn slightly and "walked" laterally along the transverse process until a paraesthesia is elicited. The **downward** direction of the needle is important as it will prevent the spinal canal being entered with consequent inadvertent spinal or epidural block.

A nerve stimulator may be used with an appropriate insulated needle (see p. 34). Muscle twitching in the arm or hand (but **not** the shoulder girdle) indicates close proximity to the nerves of the plexus.

Fig. 13.

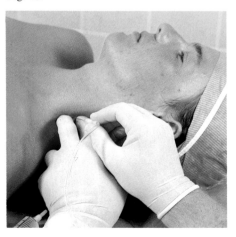

Fig. 14.

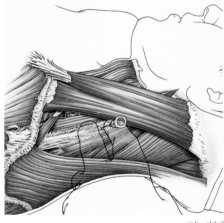

© buckhö

Injection

It is advisable to ask an assistant to make the injection using a flexible cannula so that neither the hand holding the needle nor the palpating hand need be moved during the injection (see ''Immobile needle'', p. 35). A very small amount (0.5 ml) should be injected first (after initial aspiration to eliminate the possibility of intravascular injection) and the patient questioned about any pain which would indicate a direct intraneural injection. If such pain occurs the needle should be withdrawn about 1 mm and the injection repeated. If no pain is experienced the main injection is given. The first 10 ml can be injected rapidly to elicit a dull ache in the neck, confirming the entrance of local anaesthetic into the perivascular sheath. The rest of the solution can be given more slowly, with several attempts to aspirate blood. No drug should be seen or felt to enter the subcutaneous tissues which would indicate too superficial an injection. Immediately after the injection the groove should be massaged both upwards and downwards.

Complete anaesthesia may take 30-40 min but signs of a developing block should occur within a few minutes. Tingling and a feeling of warmth in the limb are the first to appear. A sympathetic block with a warm hand and dilated veins compared to the unblocked side appears soon after. The first sign of motor block is seen in the shoulder. The distribution of the fully developed block is shown in Fig. 15. Any deficiency in the anaesthesia can be made up with supplementary blocks at the wrist or elbow.

Drugs and dose

30-40 ml of 1.5% prilocaine or 0.375% bupivacaine, or their equivalent (see p. 23). Epinephrine 1:200.000 may be added for increased effect and longer duration. Carbonated solutions give more profound blocks than hydrochlorides.

Fig. 15.

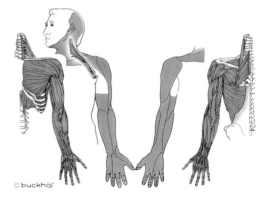

© buckhöj

Complications

Spinal or epidural blockade

This can occur if the needle is directed cephalad instead of caudad, and enters an intervertebral foramen. It may also occur in some patients with an exceptionally long dural cuff extending some distance from the intervertebral foramen.

Epidural block will be diagnosed from the relatively slow onset of bilateral anaesthesia of the neck and thorax. Hypotension may occur and should be treated with a vasopressor, and/or IV fluids; otherwise no other therapy will be required.

Spinal anaesthesia will occur rapidly and may be associated with apnoea and unconsciousness. The respiration must be assisted or controlled and the blood pressure supported until the block wears off, which may take 1-2 h depending upon the dose and drug used (see p. 72).

Acute generalised toxicity

Because a large volume and dose of drug is being used, toxicity may be a problem. Care must be taken to ensure that the recommended volume and concentration is used. If toxicity does occur, it will probably be seen 10-20 min after completing the injection. Inadvertent IV injection is unlikely, especially if frequent aspirations are made. Inadvertent intra-arterial injection, e.g. into the vertebral artery, will cause a rapid and severe reaction with convulsions after injecting only a few millilitres of solution, as the drug goes direct and undiluted to the brain. Again, arterial puncture should be easily recognised by aspiration.

Intraneural injection

Provided the initial small injection elicits the diagnosis, no permanent damage should ensue. Intraneural injection of larger amounts of drug can cause prolonged neuropathy.

Supraclavicular brachial plexus block

There are several methods of supraclavicular brachial plexus block. The one described here is the subclavian perivascular block of Winnie which is much less likely to produce pneumothorax than other techniques.

Anatomy

As the brachial plexus passes between the clavicle and the first rib, it is joined by the subclavian artery, which runs deep to the anterior scalene muscle. The three trunks of the plexus are, as their names (superior, middle and inferior) imply, in a **vertical** plane lateral to the subclavian artery (Fig. 16).

Fig. 16.

1. First rib
2. Subclavian vein
3. Subclavian artery
4. Inferior trunk
5. Middle trunk
6. Superior trunk
7. Anterior scalene muscle
8. Middle scalene muscle
9. Transverse process of C6

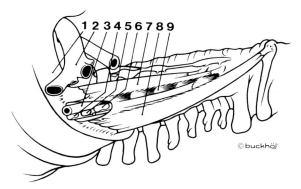

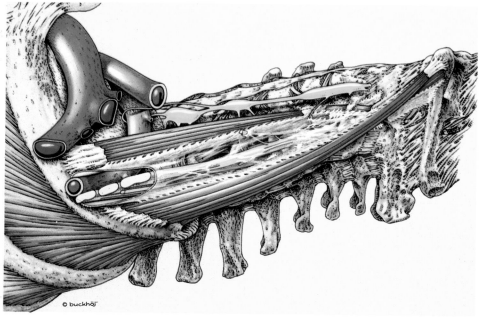

41

Patient position

Supine with arms at the side and head turned slightly away from the side to be injected. The arm on the injected side may be pulled downward to depress the clavicle and the shoulder, but the muscles should be relaxed.

Landmarks

1. Subclavian artery just above the junction of the medial and middle parts of the clavicle. Normally it can be identified by palpation of the arterial pulse. In fat or muscular necks, it is often unpalpable, but can be easily identified with an ultrasound probe (see p. 34).

2. The interscalene groove posterior to the sternomastoid muscle.

Needle insertion

The interscalene groove should be identified just above the clavicle by an index finger (the left for a left-sided block and the right for a right-sided block). The needle (4 cm, short bevelled) is inserted just above the palpating finger immediately lateral to the subclavian artery (Figs. 17 and 18). It is directed vertically downwards towards the patient's feet. It should not proceed medially, laterally or posteriorly. It is advanced slowly until a paraesthesia, **felt below the shoulder,** is obtained. If no paraesthesia is obtained, the needle will eventually contact the first rib. It should be withdrawn and the process repeated as close as possible to the artery. As long as the needle does not point backwards and medially there is no danger of penetrating the pleura. Alternatively a nerve stimulator can be used (see p. 34) with an insulated needle, and muscular twitching in the arm or hand (**not** the shoulder girdle) indicates correct placement, paraesthesia need not be elicited.

Fig. 17.

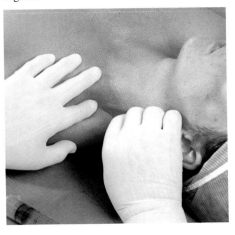

Fig. 18.

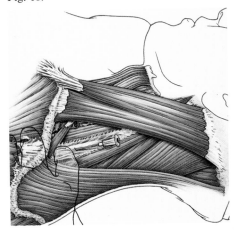

© buckhöj

Injection

Once a paraesthesia is felt, or muscular twitching elicited with the nerve stimulator, **below** the shoulder, needle advancement is stopped and the syringe and plastic extension tube attached (see p. 35) by an assistant. 0.5 ml of local anaesthetic is injected quickly. If a sudden and severe pain is felt, the needle is intraneural and must be withdrawn 1-2 mm. If no such pain occurs, the main injection is given and it frequently causes a dull aching pain ("pressure paraesthesia") confirming correct placement in the neurovascular sheath.

A sympathetic blockade causing warmth and dilated veins in the hand and arm occur within a few minutes. Motor weakness will appear in 5-10 min but it may take 20-40 min to produce full anaesthetic effect. Any deficiency in the anaesthesia can be made up with individual nerve blocks at the wrist or elbow.

Drugs and dose

30-50 ml of 1.5% lidocaine, 0.375% bupivacaine or their equivalent (see p. 23) with epinephrine 1:200.000. When larger volumes (40 ml or more) are used, the less toxic drugs prilocaine or mepivacaine are advised (see p. 24). Carbonated solutions give more profound blocks than hydrochlorides.

Complications

Arterial puncture
This indicates the needle is too anteromedial. Of itself it is not harmful, though a haematoma may occur. The needle must be withdrawn from the artery and moved more posterolateral, still keeping in the same strictly caudad direction.

Intraneural injection
Provided the initial small injection elicits the diagnosis, no permanent damage should ensue. Intraneural injection of larger amounts of drug can cause prolonged neuropathy.

Pneumothorax
Pneumothorax or accidental spinal/epidural block should not occur if the needle is correctly directed. If a large amount of air enters the pleural cavity, the classical signs and symptoms of pneumothorax will occur (p. 32). Otherwise an X-ray will be required to make the diagnosis.

Acute generalised toxicity
Acute generalised toxicity (see p. 25). Because a large volume and dose of drug is being used, toxicity may be a problem. Care must be taken to ensure the recommended volume and concentration are used. If it does occur, toxicity will probably be seen 10-20 min after completing the injection. Inadvertent IV injection is unlikely, especially if frequent aspirations are made.

Spinal/epidural block
This may occur in patients with exceptionally long dural cuffs but is much less common than with interscalene block.

Axillary brachial plexus block

Axillary block is the most commonly used method of brachial plexus block, probably because it is not associated with pneumothorax. Unless large volumes are injected, it is less likely to anaesthetise the shoulder than the other methods.

Anatomy

After passing from the neck between the clavicle and first rib, the brachial plexus enters the upper limb via the axilla (Fig. 19). At this point the trunks of the plexus have each divided into an anterior and a posterior division which combine to form the three cords, lateral, medial and posterior. All the nerves are in close relationship to the axillary artery and lie within the perivascular sheath. In the lower axilla, the trunks divide and form the four main terminal branches, the median, radial, ulnar and musculocutaneous nerves. The last mentioned quickly leaves the perivascular sheath through the coracobrachialis muscle.

Patient position

The upper limb on the injected side should be abducted at the shoulder and flexed at right angles at the elbow so that the wrist is at the same level as the patient's head. The hand should not be **under** the head, as this compresses the structures as they pass close to the coracoid process.

Landmarks

The axillary artery should be palpated and followed as high up into the axilla as possible. If the arterial pulsation is difficult to feel, ultrasound will accurately identify the artery (see p. 34).

Fig. 19.

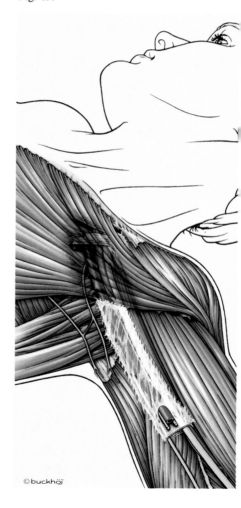

© buckhöj

Needle insertion

A 4-cm short bevelled needle, attached to a plastic extension tube, is used. If a nerve stimulator is to be used, an insulated needle is preferred (see p. 34). The axillary artery is palpated continuously and the needle inserted just above the artery. It is directed towards the apex of the axilla, i.e. in almost the same plane as the neuromuscular bundle (Figs. 20 and 21). The needle is advanced slowly, keeping close to the artery until a paraesthesia is felt, or twitching of muscles in the arm or hand is seen with a nerve stimulator (see p. 34). Penetration of the neurovascular sheath is usually felt as a definite "give" as the needle is advanced. If the needle is then left untouched, it will be seen to move with each arterial beat, confirming its close relationship to the artery.

If the needle enters the artery it may be withdrawn and realigned. Some authorities enter the artery on purpose, the needle being directed at right angles to the artery. When arterial blood is seen, the needle is advanced so as to exit the artery opposite its entry point, where it will be within the perivascular sheath.

It should be possible to insert a catheter through the needle and into the perivascular sheath. There should be no obstruction to the forward movement of the catheter if the needle is correctly placed.

Fig. 20.

Fig. 21.

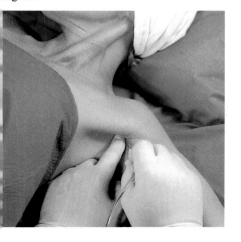

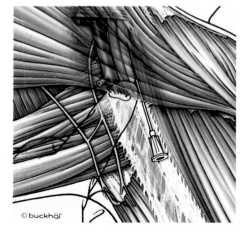

Injection

Using an assistant, the syringe is attached to the extension tube and if aspiration of blood is negative, 0.5 ml is injected. Acute severe pain following this indicates an intraneural injection and the needle must be withdrawn 1-2 mm. If no pain occurs, the main injection should be given. Little or no resistance to the injection should be encountered. It may cause a dull ache due to pressure within the perivascular sheath. To encourage the local anaesthetic solution to travel upwards in the sheath and not downwards, the palpating finger is pressed firmly on the artery distal to the needle during and after the injection.

A sympathetic blockade causing warmth and dilated veins in the hand and arm occurs within a few minutes. Motor weakness will appear in 5-10 min but it may take 20-40 min to produce the full effect. The distribution of the fully developed block is shown in Fig. 22. Any deficiency in the anaesthesia can be made up with individual nerve blocks at the wrist or elbow.

Fig. 22.

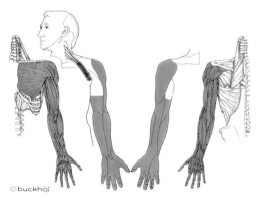

© buckhöj

Drugs and dose

30-40 ml of 1.5% lidocaine or 0.375% bupivacaine or their equivalent (see p. 23) with epinephrine 1:200.000. With the larger volumes, prilocaine or mepivacaine are to be preferred on account of their lower toxicity.

Carbonated solutions give more profound blocks than hydrochlorides.

Complications

Acute generalised toxicity

Acute generalised toxicity (see p. 25). Because a large volume and dose of drug is being used, toxicity may be a problem. Care must be taken to ensure the recommended volume and concentration are used. If it does occur, toxicity will probably be seen 10-20 min after completing the injection. Inadvertent IV injection is unlikely, especially if frequent aspirations are made, but if it occurs overt toxicity will be seen within a few minutes.

Intraneural injection

Provided the initial small injection elicit the diagnosis, no permanent damage should ensue. Intraneural injection of larger amounts of drug can cause prolonged neuropathy.

Digital nerve block of the finger

This is a simple and effective way of anaesthetising a finger.

Anatomy

Two digital nerves run on each side of each finger, a palmar and a dorsal branch (Fig. 23).

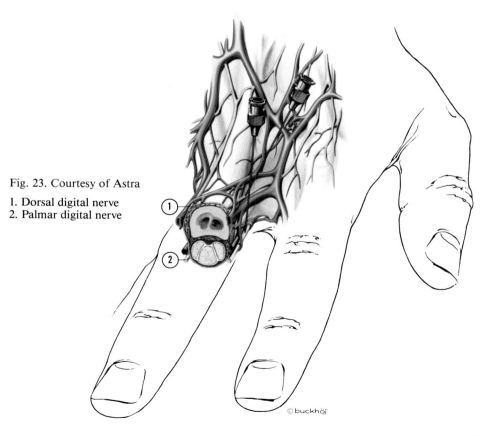

Fig. 23. Courtesy of Astra

1. Dorsal digital nerve
2. Palmar digital nerve

Needle insertion

The easiest method is to insert a needle at the base of the digit to contact the proximal phalanx at its lateral point (Fig. 24). Withdraw the needle fractionally and deposit 0.5 ml of local anaesthetic. Redirect the needle towards the dorsal part of the digit (Fig. 25) and inject a further 1 ml as the needle is slowly withdrawn. Repeating this on the palmar aspect of the digit (Fig. 26) will leave a semicircle of local anaesthetic. When repeated on the other side of the digit, a complete ring of the injected drug, will surround the base of the finger.

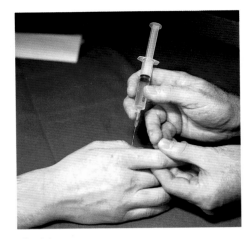

Fig. 24.a.

Fig. 24.b. The digital nerves of the finger.

1. Dorsal digital nerve

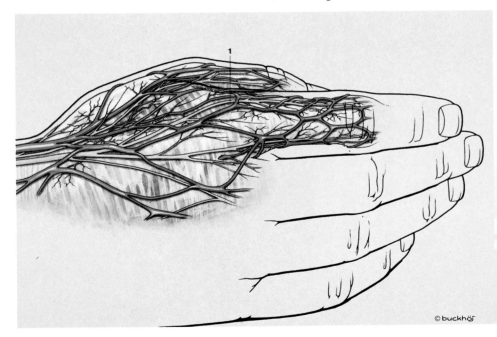

© buckhöj

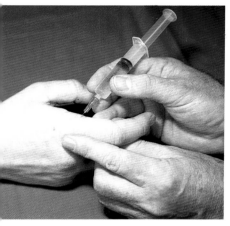

Fig. 25.

Alternatively the injection can be made proximal to the base of the digit to block the nerves as they run between the metacarpal bones. The needle is inserted 2 cm proximal to the web of the digit until it is within the space between the adjacent bones (Fig. 27). Inject 1 ml while withdrawing slowly. By palpating the space as the injection is made, the filling of the space will be felt. An intercarpal injection anaesthetises the adjacent sides of

Fig. 26.

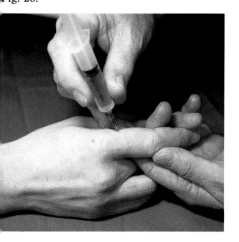

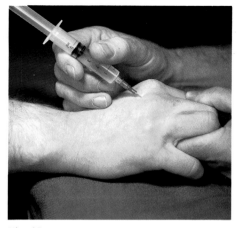

Fig. 27.

two digits and therefore to complete the anaesthesia of a whole digit the adjacent space must also be injected with 3 ml (Fig. 28).

Drugs and dose

4 ml of lidocaine 1% or its equivalent (see p. 23). Epinephrine is not recommended in digital blocks.

Fig. 28.

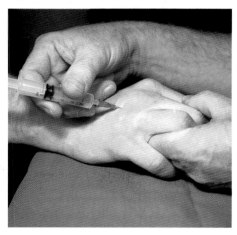

Lower limb

The lower limb can be rendered anaesthetic simply and effectively by spinal or epidural block. However, these techniques involve some degree of sympathetic blockade and there may be patients in whom this should be avoided. As with the upper limb, the nerves to the lower limb can be blocked at any part of their course from the spine to the periphery. The three main nerves are the sciatic, the femoral and the obturator nerves. The lateral cutaneous nerve of thigh is smaller and supplies skin only. They all derive from the lumbar and sacral plexuses. The lumbar plexus (L2, 3, 4) gives rise to the femoral and obturator nerves and also to the lateral cutaneous nerve of the thigh. The lumbar plexus lies in the posterior part of the psoas muscle. The sacral plexus (L4, 5, S1, 2, 3 and 4) gives rise to the sciatic nerve. The sciatic nerve leaves the pelvis through the greater sciatic foramen and enters the back of the thigh between the greater trochanter of the femur and the tuberosity of the ischium. It divides, in the lower third of the posterior thigh, into its two main terminal branches, the tibial and common peroneal nerves.

The cutaneous distribution of the three largest nerves is shown in Fig. 29. All three nerves supply both the hip and the knee joints and to obtain complete anaesthesia of the lower limb it is necessary to block all three. A femoral nerve block by itself is effective in relieving the pain of a fractured shaft of femur, but not of the femoral neck. Block of the lateral cutaneous nerve of thigh alone allows skin grafts to be taken from the lateral thigh.

Fig. 29.

■ Sciatic nerve
■ Femoral nerve
■ Obturator nerve

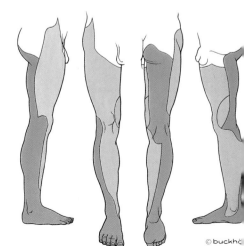

© buckhé

Sciatic nerve block

The sciatic nerve is the biggest nerve in the body but it lies deep in the posterior thigh. There are three main approaches to the nerve, anterior with the patient lying supine, posterior with the patient in the lateral position and posterior with the patient supine and the hip and knee joint flexed to right angles as in the lithotomy position (Raj approach). The choice will depend upon the ability to turn the patient appropriately without discomfort, e.g. for patients with fractured bones, the anterior approach is best. Whichever method is used, a nerve stimulator technique is strongly advised (see p. 34).

Anterior sciatic approach

This is particularly suitable for patients lying supine who cannot be turned laterally or have their hip and knee joints flexed, e.g. those with fractures.

Anatomy

While the sciatic nerve for much of its course lies behind the femur, it is medial to the bone at the level of the lesser trochanter and is therefore accessible to a needle inserted anteriorly.

Fig. 30.

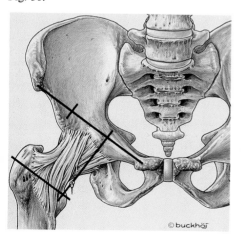

Fig. 31.
Courtesy
of
Astra.

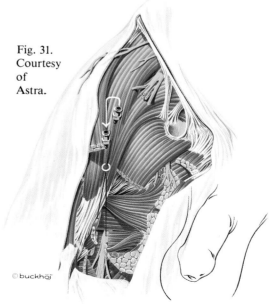

Patient position

Supine

Landmarks

1. Anterior superior iliac spine
2. Pubic tubercle
3. Greater trochanter

Draw a line from the anterior superior iliac spine to the pubic tubercle along the inguinal ligament, and a parallel line from the greater trochanter across the upper thigh. Connect the two parallel lines with a line at right angles to both from the junction of the medial and middle thirds of the upper line. The point where the connecting line joins the lower line marks the position of the lesser trochanter (Fig. 30).

Fig. 32.

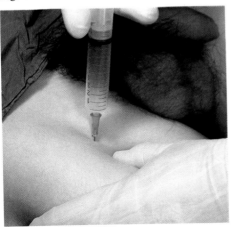

Needle insertion

The usual description of the anterior approach advises needle insertion directly over the point marking the lesser trochanter. However, long needles bend easily, and often contacting the femoral shaft it is not easy to redirect towards the sciatic nerve. A more medial insertion is therefore advisable. A long (12-15 cm) needle is inserted perpendicularly downwards through the skin **1 cm medial** to the point which marks the position of the lesser trochanter (Fig. 31).

Push the needle in a vertical direction (with the patient supine) and slightly laterally to contact the lesser trochanter or shaft of the femur (Fig. 32). Withdraw almost to the skin and realign until the needle passes medially to the femur. The sciatic nerve will be found about 5 cm behind the femur. Using a nerve stimulator observe the foot for movement during stimulation. The needle point is adjusted to the optimal position (see p. 34).

Drugs and dose

15-20 ml of 1.5% lidocaine or 0.375% bupivacaine (or their equivalent, see p. 23). Epinephrine 1:200.000 may be added. If this nerve block is being combined with a femoral 3 in 1 block, then quite large amounts of local anaesthetic may need to be injected. In such cases prilocaine 1.5% is the drug of choice due to its low toxicity. As the two injections will be separated by an interval of several minutes, the danger of toxicity will be considerably reduced.

Complications

1. Acute toxicity (see p. 25).
2. Intraneural injection with neuropathy (see p. 31).

Posterior approach

Anatomy

The sciatic nerve leaves the pelvis through the greater sciatic foramen and may be blocked just inferior to this, as it passes below the piriformis muscle.

Patient position

Lateral with side to be injected uppermost. The thigh and knee are flexed at right angles so that the limb lies in front of the dependent limb.

Landmarks

1. Greater trochanter
2. Posterior superior iliac spine

Join these with a line and draw a second line at right angles from its midpoint (Fig. 33).

Needle insertion

The needle should be inserted at a point 4 cm down the second line, through the gluteus maximus (Fig. 33). It is advanced slowly until the nerve stimulator causes movement of the foot, usually about 7-8 cm from the skin. The needle point is adjusted to the optimal position (see p. 34).

Drugs and dose

15-20 ml of 1.5% lidocaine or 0.375% bupivacaine (or their equivalent, see p. 23). Epinephrine 1:200.000 may be added. If this nerve block is being combined with a femoral 3 in 1 block, then quite large amounts of local anaesthetic may need to be injected. In such cases prilocaine 1.5% is the drug of choice due to its low toxicity. As the two injections will be separated by an interval of several minutes, the danger of toxicity will be considerably reduced.

Complications

1. Acute toxicity (see p. 25)
2. Intraneural injection with neuropathy (see p. 31)

Fig. 33. Courtesy of Astra.

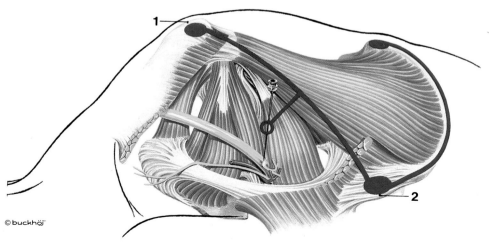

© buckhöj

Posterior approach, Raj technique

Anatomy

In this approach the patient remains supine, but the lower limb is raised into the lithotomy position. In this position the sciatic nerve is stretched and therefore more firmly fixed as it passes between the greater trochanter and the ischial tuberosity. The nerve is thus blocked a little lower than in the classical posterior approach.

Patient position

Supine with the lower limb in the lithotomy position (hip and knee flexed to right angles). The limb may be held by an assistant (Fig. 34).

Landmarks

1. Greater trochanter
2. Ischial tuberosity

Needle insertion

The needle is inserted at right angles to the skin at the midpoint between the greater trochanter and the ischial tuberosity. It is advanced until the nerve stimulator causes movement of the foot, and the needle point is in the optimal position (see p. 34).

Drugs and dose

15-20 ml of 1.5% lidocaine or 0.375% bupivacaine (or their equivalent, see p. 23). Epinephrine 1:200.000 may be added. If this nerve block is being combined with a femoral 3 in 1 block, then quite large amounts of local anaesthetic may need to be injected. In such cases prilocaine 1.5% is the drug of choice due to its low toxicity. As the two injections will be separated by an interval of several minutes, the danger of toxicity will be considerably reduced.

Complications

1. Acute toxicity (see p. 25)
2. Intraneural injection with neuropathy (see p. 31)

Fig. 34.a.

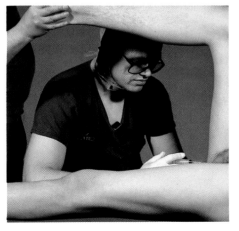

Fig. 34.b.

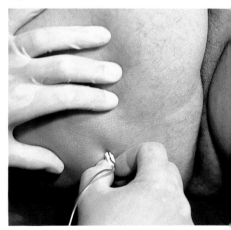

3 in 1 lumbar plexus block

This block anaesthetises the femoral, obturator and lateral cutaneous nerve of the thigh. When combined with a sciatic block, the entire lower limb is effected.

Anatomy

The lumbar plexus lies in the posterior part of the psoas muscle. The quadratus lumborum and iliacus muscles lie posteriorly. Like the brachial plexus, the lumbar plexus is enclosed within a sheath of connective tissue which can be entered at the level of the inguinal ligament where the femoral nerve enters the thigh (Fig. 35).

Local anaesthetic injected at this point will spread cephalad between the iliacus and psoas muscles, blocking all the branches of the lumbar plexus.

Patient position

Supine.

Landmarks

1. Inguinal ligament
2. Femoral artery

Fig. 35. Courtesy of Astra.

1. Lateral cutaneous nerve of the thigh
2. Femoral nerve

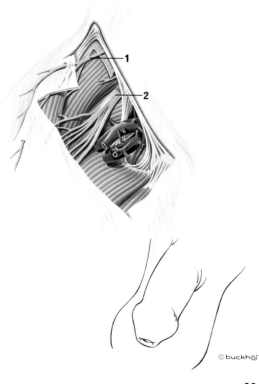

© buckhöj

Needle insertion

The needle is inserted just below the inguinal ligament, 1-1.5 cm lateral to the femoral artery (Fig. 36). The needle is directed cephalad at about 60° from the skin, and advanced slowly until either a paraesthesia is elicited or a nerve stimulator causes movement of the patella.

Drugs and dose

25-30 ml of 1.5% lidocaine or 0.375% bupivacaine, or their equivalent (see p. 23). Epinephrine 1:200.000 can be added. If combined with sciatic nerve block, prilocaine 1-5% or mepivacaine 1.5% are recommended because of their lower toxicity. As the two injections will be separated by an interval of several minutes, the danger of toxicity will be considerably reduced.

Complications

1. Acute toxicity (see p. 25)
2. Neuropathy due to intraneural injection (see p. 31)

Femoral nerve block

This is a particularly good block for patients with a fracture of the shaft of the femur as it allows painless reduction of the fracture and the application of the traction.

The technique is exactly the same as for the 3 in 1 block but less drug, 10-15 ml, is used.

Fig. 36.

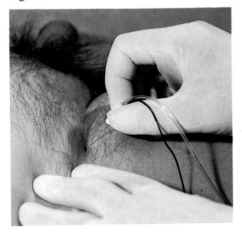

Digital nerve block of the toe

This is a simple and effective way of anaesthetising a toe.

Anatomy

Two nerves run on either side of each toe, a plantar and a dorsal digital nerve (Fig. 37).

Fig. 37.
1. Superficial peroneal nerve
2. Deep peroneal nerve
3. Dorsal digital nerve
4. Plantar digital nerve

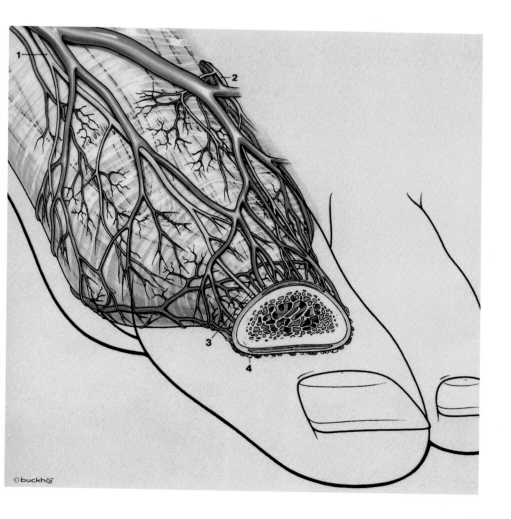

© buckhöj

Needle insertion

The easiest method is to insert a needle at the base of the digit to contact the proximal phalanx at its lateral point (Fig. 38). Withdraw the needle fractionally and deposit 0.5 ml of local anaesthetic. Redirect the needle towards the dorsal part of the digit (Fig. 39) and inject a further 1 ml as the needle is slowly withdrawn. Repeating this on the plantar aspect of the digit (Fig. 40) will leave a semicircle of local anaesthetic which, when repeated on the other side of the digit, will surround the base of the finger with a complete ring of the injected drug.

Drugs and dose

4 ml of lidocaine 1% ml or its equivalent (see p. 23). Epinephrine is not recommended in digital blocks.

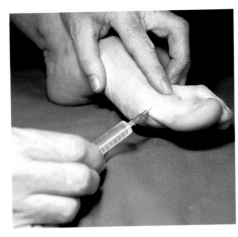

Fig. 39.

Fig. 38.

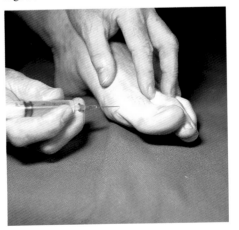

Fig. 40.

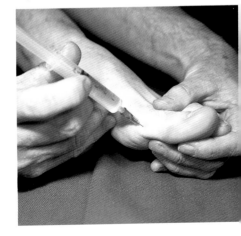

Intravenous regional anaesthesia (Bier's block)

Intravenous regional anaesthesia is a simple and effective method of producing anaesthesia of the limbs, both upper and lower. It is based on the fact that if the circulation to a limb is occluded and an injection of local anaesthetic is made into a vein distal to that occlusion, the drug will reach the capillaries by retrograde flow and enter the extravascular space. Here it will come into contact with nerve endings and nerve trunks, causing numbness and paralysis of the limb below the tourniquet for the duration of the circulatory occlusion.

Method

Upper limb

1. All drugs, oxygen and equipment necessary for the treatment of toxicity should be available (Fig.41). Venous access in the non-operated limb should be established.

2. An inflatable tourniquet is placed around the upper arm over a wool bandage to protect the skin. Ideally, the tourniquet should be one specially designed for the purpose with a gauge and hand pump (Fig. 42a).

Alternatively, an ordinary sphygmomanometer cuff may be used if essential precautions are taken. It must be very carefully tested for leaks and the connection to the mercury column or pressure gauge must be totally secure. Once the cuff is pressurised, it is vital that deflation

Fig. 41.

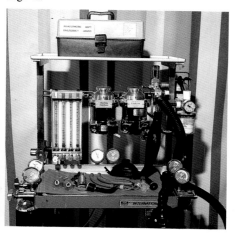

Fig. 42 a and b.

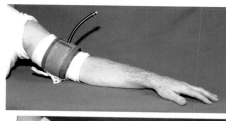

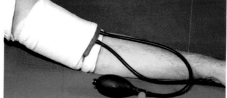

below arterial pressure does not occur accidentally. To prevent sudden deflation due to slipping of the cuff, a non-elastic bandage should be wrapped around the cuff (Fig. 42b).

3. A needle, a 23 gauge butterfly needle or a small IV plastic cannula (Fig. 43), is placed into a vein on the dorsum of the hand and secured to the skin.

4. The limb is exsanguinated of venous blood. This may be done by applying an Esmarch or elastic bandage from the hand up to the blood pressure cuff (Fig. 44). In cases of fractures when this process may be painful, the limb may simply be raised vertical for a few minutes to empty the veins as much as possible, without applying the bandage (Fig. 45).

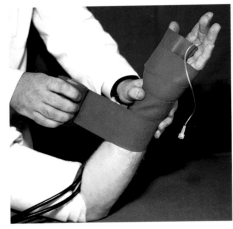

Fig. 44.

Fig. 43.

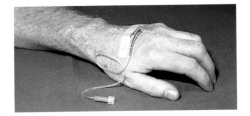

Fig. 45.

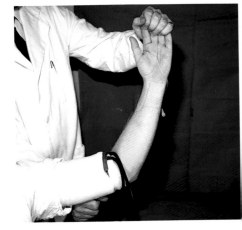

5. The blood pressure cuff is then inflated to 250 mmHg or 100 mmHg above systolic pressure, and the Esmarch or elastic bandage below the cuff removed (Fig. 46).

6. Local anaesthetic is now injected into the indwelling needle. This injection should be slow, not exceeding 1 ml every 2 s. The drug will be seen to enter the capillaries and produce pale areas of skin (Fig. 47).

7. At least 10-15 min must be allowed to achieve anaesthesia before beginning the surgical procedure (Fig. 48).

8. Following the completion of surgery, and not within 20 min of completing the local anaesthetic injection, the blood pressure cuff may be deflated. Reactive hyperaemia will be observed (Fig.49). The longer the tourniquet is in place, the more local anaesthetic will reach the extracellular space, reducing the amount of drug which will be released on removal of the tourniquet.

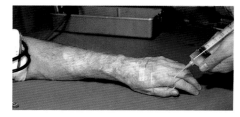

Fig. 47.

9. Normal sensation and muscle function will return within a few minutes, though patchy anaesthesia may remain for up to 60 min.

Fig. 46.

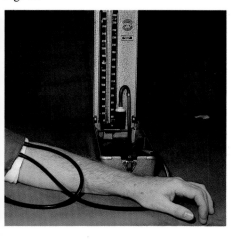

Fig. 48.

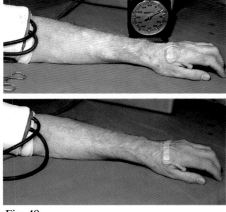

Fig. 49.

61

Drugs and dose

40 ml is usually required in an adult though this should be reduced in children (0.5 ml/kg body weight) or if the limb is clearly small and thin. The solution must be dilute, i.e. 0.5% of prilocaine, lidocaine or mepivacaine. Other agents such as bupivacaine are not recommended nor should epinephrine be added. Remember the drug is being injected intravenously and toxicity can easily occur with accidental deflation of the cuff. Too rapid an injection can produce a high pressure within the veins and drug can escape past the tourniquet. This may also occure if veins are not emtied before injection.

Lower limb

For lower limb surgery the tourniquet cuff may be placed on the thigh, the calf or the ankle depending upon the site of the operation. An intravenous needle or cannula is placed in a vein on the dorsum of the foot. After exsanguinating the limb, the cuff should be inflated to a pressure of 300 mmHg or at least 150 mmHg above the systolic pressure (Fig. 50a). The procedure is thereafter the same as for the upper limb.

Drugs and dose

With a thigh cuff the dose is 40-60 ml of dilute local anaesthetic, 0.5% prilocaine, lidocaine or mepivacaine. With a calf (Fig. 50b) or ankle (Fig. 51) tourniquet the dose is 30 or 20 ml respectively.

Fig. 50 a and b.

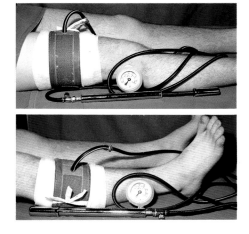

Fig. 51.

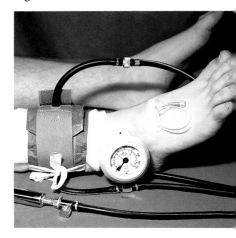

Complications

Toxicity

This may be due to accidental deflation of the cuff during or soon after injection of the local anaesthetic. Drug may also pass beneath the inflated tourniquet and reach the systemic circulation during the injection if the limb is not properly exsanguinated before inflating the cuff, and/or the injection is made too rapidly. Both can raise the pressure in the veins to levels above the pressure in the cuff. The signs, symptoms and treatment of toxicity are given on p. 25-27.

Tourniquet pain

After 20 min or so the inflated tourniquet cuff may become very painful. If a second cuff is placed distal to the original one the tissues beneath it will be anaesthetised. The second cuff may then be inflated painlessly. Once the second cuff has been secured and inflated, the first one may be deflated. Specially designed double cuffs are available.

Intercostal nerve block

This is a simple block to perform and has uses both by itself and in conjunction with general anaesthesia. Usually several intercostal nerves must be blocked. The main indications are:

Fig. 52.
1. Intercostal nerve (ventral ramus)
2. Lateral cutaneous branch
3. Anterior cutaneous branch
4. Endothoracic fascia
5. Intercostalis externus muscle
6. Intercostalis internus muscle
7. Intercostalis intimus muscle

1. To provide postoperative pain relief after abdominal surgery, especially if the incision is unilateral, e.g. Kocher's incision for cholecystectomy. The 7th to 11th intercostal nerves are blocked on the appropriate side.
2. To provide postoperative pain relief after thoracotomy. In these cases the nerves may be blocked under direct vision from **within** the thorax.

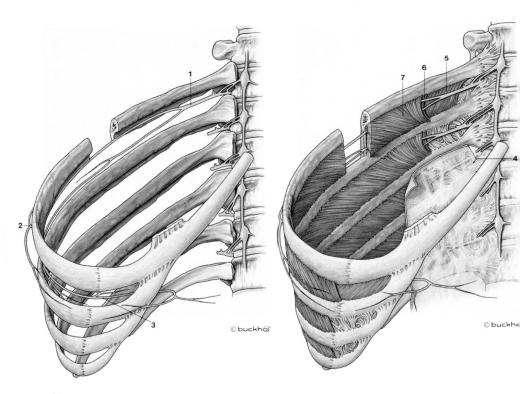

© buckhöj

© buckh

3. To relieve the pain of fractured ribs. This can also assist in the treatment as it allows greater respiratory movement and painless coughing. The appropriate nerves are blocked posterior to the fractures.

4. To provide muscular relaxation and analgesia in conjunction with light general anaesthesia in abdominal surgery. In such cases the patient will be intubated but may be allowed to breathe spontaneously.

Anatomy

Each intercostal nerve derives from the ventral ramus of the corresponding thoracic spinal nerve. These pass laterally from the paravertebral space to reach the inferior border of the ribs. They run at first between the pleura and the posterior intercostal fascia but soon reach the space between the intercostalis internus and intimus muscles. Here they divide into two or more branches which run in the intercostal spaces supplying the muscles and skin of the thorax and abdomen. At the midaxillary line they each give off a lateral cutaneous branch which supplies the skin of the posterolateral parts of the thorax and abdomen (Fig. 52).

The upper six nerves terminate at the sternum and their branches supply the skin of the anterior part of the thorax. The lower six nerves pass under the costal margin and supply the muscles and skin of the anterior abdominal wall. The lateral cutaneous branches pierce the intercostalis externus and divide into anterior and posterior branches to supply the skin of the lateral wall of the abdomen (as far forward as the lateral border of the rectus muscle) and the back respectively.

The cutaneous branches of the intercostal nerves communicate freely with adjacent nerves, leading to overlapping of the nerve supply. However, the major part of the skin and musculature of the abdominal wall can be anaesthetised by blockade of the 6th to 12th intercostal nerves.

In recent years there has been considerable controversy on whether there was intercommunication between adjacent intercostal spaces. At their origin the intercostal nerves, lie between the pleura and the posterior intercostal fascia and there is nothing to stop local anaesthetic spreading extrapleurally and affecting several adjacent nerves. Even when injected laterally at or near the costal angle, drug can reach the extrapleural space. This is made easier if ribs are fractured, when even subpleural spread can occur. These factors have led to the use of a single large volume injection in the intercostal space with the intention of causing blockade of several nerves. While this may be useful with multiple fractured ribs, the spread is unpredictable and it is better to give multiple small volume injections at the appropriate intercostal spaces.

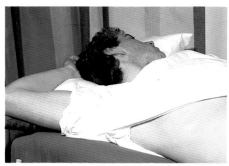

Fig. 53.

Patient position

1. Supine for blocks in the midaxillary line. This is by far the most convenient position. The arm is raised with the hand behind the head exposing the lateral thoracic wall (Fig.53). Right-handed anaesthetists should face the patient's feet while blocking the right sided nerves (Fig. 54) and face the patient's head for the left sided nerves (Fig. 55). (Vice versa for left-handed anaesthetists.)
2. Lateral for unilateral blocks at the angle of the ribs.
3. Prone for bilateral blocks at the angle of the ribs.

Landmarks

1. The ribs, counting upwards from the 12th
2. The costal angles, 7-10 cm from the midline posteriorly
3. The midaxillary line

The nerves to be blocked will be determined by the indication for the block. For fractured ribs the local anaesthetic is placed close to the rib proximal to the fracture. With multiple blocks for post-operative pain relief (or as an adjunct to general anaesthesia) in abdominal surgery, the classical site for injection is at the angle of the rib, which involves the patient being in the lateral or prone (if the block is to be bilateral) position. However, drug injected into the intercostal spaces has been shown to run backwards and forwards in the spaces for several centimetres. Thus if the midaxillary line is used, the intercostal nerves, including their lateral branches, are easily blocked and the patient can remain supine.

Fig. 54.

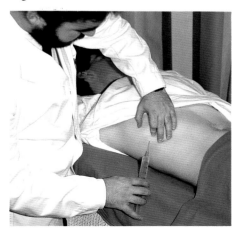

Fig. 55.

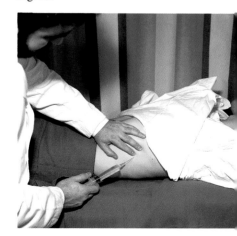

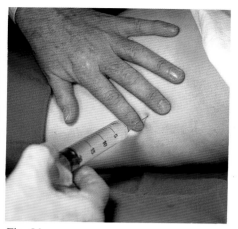

Fig. 56.

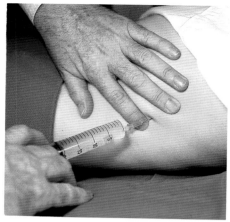

Fig. 58.

Needle insertion

Regardless of the site of injection (mid-axillary or angle of the rib), the technique of needle insertion is the same. The needle point should be in close proximation to the rib if puncture of the pleura is to be avoided.

The rib is held between the second and third fingers of the non-dominant hand. The needle, attached to a syringe, is inserted between the fingers and advanced to contact the rib (Fig. 56). The needle should be directed towards the rib but tilted 20° (Fig. 57a) cephalad. The needle is then "walked" down the rib until it

Fig. 57 a-c.

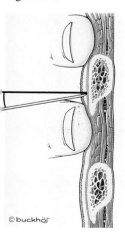
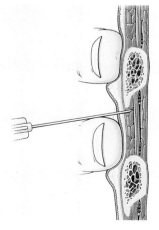
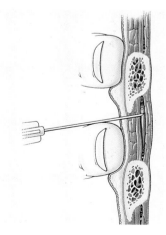

© buckhöj

slides under the rib, still maintaining the cephalad direction (Fig. 57b). It is advanced 3 mm deep to the external surface of the rib (Figs. 57c and 58). The anaesthetist will feel a "click" as the intercostalis externa is pierced and the needle will reach the space between internus and intimus. 2-3 ml of local anaesthetic is injected. (An alternative method is to angle the needle almost in the plane of the rib so as to reduce the risk of pleural puncture.)

Drugs and dose

2% lidocaine, 0.5% bupivacaine or their equivalent. Epinephrine 1:200.000 may be added. Use 2-3 ml per nerve. Maximum dose 20-25 ml.

Complications

Pneumothorax

To cause a pneumothorax the needle must penetrate the pleura **and** puncture the lung itself, thus allowing sufficient air to escape into the pleural cavity and collapse the lung. Coughing and positive pressure respiration will increase the volume of air in the pleural cavity if the lung is penetreted.

Provided the needle is kept in close proximity to the rib, pneumothorax is very uncommon.

Toxicity

Intercostal block gives rise to the highest plasma concentrations of local anaesthetic of the commonly used methods of regional anaesthesia. Care should therefore be taken in calculating the dose and using the appropriate drugs. Fortunately multiple bilateral blocks requiring high dosage are usually performed during a concomitant general anaesthesia and overt toxicity is unlikely. With conscious patients, the injections can be spaced out in time, e.g. over 10-15 min, and this will greatly reduce the possibility of toxicity. The diagnosis and treatment of toxicity is given on p. 25-27.

Spinal anaesthesia

Spinal anaesthesia is one of the oldest and most valuable of the techniques of regional anaesthesia. It is the most efficient of blocks, in that a small quantity of local anaesthetic injected into the spinal subarachnoid space will cause a widespread blockade of the spinal nerves. Systemic toxicity is therefore never a problem. However, though simple to perform, it does require a degree of understanding and training if it is to be used safely.

Anatomy

The spinal subarachnoid space communicates superiorly with the pontine cistern and the cerebello-medullary cistern. It is situated between the pia and arachnoid maters and contains the cerebrospinal fluid (CSF), the spinal cord, the spinal nerves and the blood vessels supplying these structures. The arachnoid mater is closely applied, but not attached, to the dura mater (Fig. 59).

The subarachnoid space ends at the level of the second sacral vertebra.

The CSF is produced in the cerebral ventricles by the choroid plexuses. It circulates through the ventricular system and into the cerebral and spinal subarachnoid space. It is absorbed back into the blood through the arachnoid villi in the superior sagittal sinus and some of the other venous sinuses. The CSF in the spinal canal has little or no active circulation and drugs injected into it will spread mainly by diffusion before being absorbed into capillaries in the pia mater, the spinal nerves and the spinal cord.

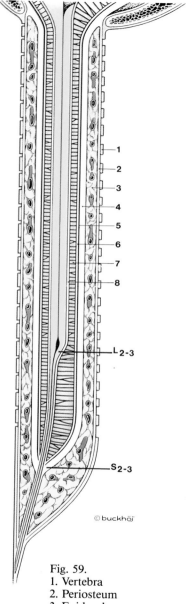

© buckhöj

Fig. 59.
1. Vertebra
2. Periosteum
3. Epidural space
4. Dura mater
5. Subdural space
6. Arachnoid mater
7. Subarachnoid space
8. Pia mater

69

Spinal nerves supply specific dermatomes in the body (Fig. 60) and different upper levels of block are required for different operations as follows:

Upper abdominal	T5 - 6
Lower abdominal	T8 - 9
Lower limb	T12
Perineal	S1
Bladder	T10
Kidney	T8

The spinal subarachnoid space is usually entered in the lumbar region (lumbar puncture), i.e. below the tip of the spinal cord. To reach the space, the needle must traverse the skin and subcutaneous tissue, the supraspinous ligament, the intraspinous ligament, the ligamentum flavum, the dura mater and the arachnoid mater.

Equipment

Spinal anaesthesia should always be carried out with full aseptic and antiseptic precautions.

Spinal needles

Spinal needles are supplied with stylets and the most commonly used vary from 22-26 French gauge. The smaller the bore of the needle, the less risk there is of post-lumbar puncture headache. Only the 22 gauge can be inserted reliably without the aid of an introducer. Thinner needles bend too easily and most of the penetration of the ligaments must be done with a short stout introducer through which the spinal needle can be inserted before the final penetration into the subarachnoid space. Disposable needles are available and a 25 gauge will easily pass through a short (4-cm) 18 gauge hypodermic needle.

Spinal pack

The spinal pack should also include:

1. Sterile drapes
2. Lotion bowel for antiseptic
3. 2-ml and 5-ml syringes
4. Needle for aspirating local anaesthetic from its ampoule
5. Ampoule of local anaesthetic
   Though some drugs can be autoclaved repeatedly, it is better that this is only done once. Ampoules in sterile packages are also available and can be "dropped" aseptically onto the sterile trolley. In drawing up solution from an ampoule, care must be taken to avoid glass fragments entering the syringe. This can be done by not "grounding" the aspiration needle on the bottom of the ampoule, or by using a filter.
6. Swabs

Patient position

1. Lateral with the spine maximally flexed by raising the knees and flexing the neck and thorax.

2. Sitting with spine maximally flexed by resting the feet on a stool and bending the trunk forward towards thighs.

If flexion is limited, either the paramedian (lateral) approach to the lumbar interspaces or a lumbosacral approach may be used.

Landmarks

Lumbar spinous processes. The iliac crest is at the level of the fourth lumbar vertebra.

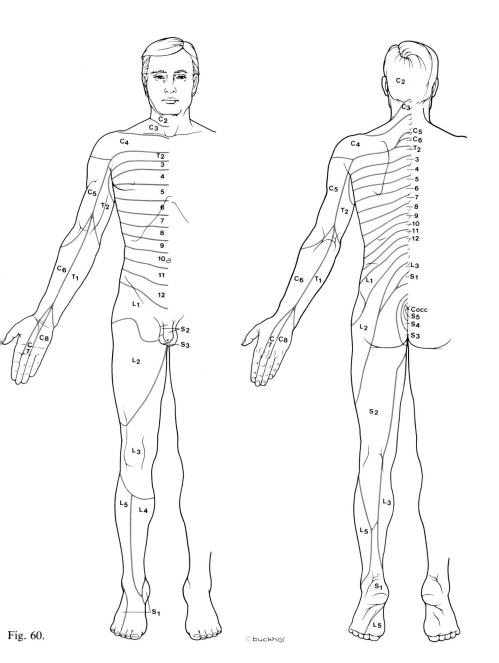

Fig. 60.

© buckhöj

71

Drugs and dose

Virtually all local anaesthetics can and have been used for spinal anaesthesia. They may be divided into:

1. Short acting (1-1 ½ h):
   lidocaine, mepivacaine, procaine

2. Medium/long acting (1 ½-4 h):
   tetracaine, bupivacaine, cinchocaine

Duration is considerably affected by dosage.

Drugs used for spinal anaesthesia are also categorised by their specific gravity (S.G.) in relation to that of the CSF, which is around 1003 at 37°C.

There is considerable confusion regarding specific gravities because these change considerably in the temperature range from 18-37° C. Thus a solution which is hyperbaric at room temperature may become hypobaric when it has warmed to body temperature. In practice there seems to be little difference in the behaviour of so-called isobaric and hypobaric solutions, both of which are largely unaffected by gravity, i.e. by the patient's posture during and after injection. Hypobaric solutions are perforce of low concentration and have often to be used in larger volumes. They will therefore take longer to reach 37°C and during this time they will be iso- or hyperbaric. It is not possible to make solutions markedly "lighter" than CSF but it is easy to make them much heavier.

Hyperbaric solutions are made by the addition of glucose 5-9%, giving an S.G. of 1020-1030.

They are affected by gravity after injection and are also less miscible with CSF. In patients kept horizontal throughout, they tend to spread more cephalad than isobaric solutions.

The most commonly employed drugs are:

Lidocaine

Available as a 5% solution in 7.5% glucose (hyperbaric). Dose 1-3 ml. Also effective as a 2% plain solution (isobaric), in a dose of 3-6 ml.

Mepivacaine

Available as 4% solution in 9.5% glucose (hyperbaric). Dose 1-3 ml. Also effective as a 2% plain solution (isobaric), in a dose of 3-6 ml.

Procaine

Usually supplied in solid crystalline form which dissolves in CSF. Procaine solutions over 2.5% concentration are hyperbaric. Dose 100-200 mg.

Tetracaine

This is available as a 1% solution which may be diluted to 0.5% with 10% glucose (hyperbaric), normal saline (isobaric) or water (hypobaric). It is also supplied as a crystalline powder which may be dissolved in CSF. The dose is 1-4 ml (5-20 mg of the powder).

Bupivacaine

Available as 0.5% in 8% glucose (hyperbaric) or as the plain 0.5% solution (isobaric). Dose 2-4 ml. In the USA 0.75% in 8.25% glucose is available (hypobaric). Dose 1-2 ml.

Cinchocaine (Dibucaine)

Available as 0.5% in 6% glucose (hyperbaric). Dose 2-3 ml. Also supplied as a hypobaric solution, 0.067% in buffered saline, dose 5-10 ml.

Midline approach

Having identified the appropriate intervertebral space, the skin is held firmly against the adjacent spinous process while the needle or introducer is directed in a slightly cephalad direction in the midline, so as to pass equidistant between the spinous processes. The bevel should be pointing laterally. No infiltration of the skin is necessary if a fine needle or a sharp introducer is used. The increased resistance of the ligamentum flavum is often felt. When it is thought that the spinal canal has been entered, the stylet is withdrawn and the needle hub examined for CSF leakage.

If an introducer is used (Fig. 61), it should only be inserted as far as the ligamentum flavum, i.e. when it is firmly engaged in the ligaments (Fig. 62). Even a short introducer can reach and pierce the dura mater in some patients, increasing the risk of headache.

Fig. 61.

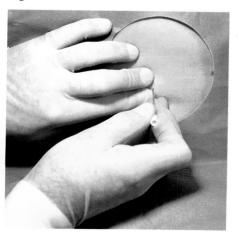

Fig. 62.

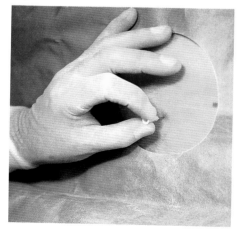

Once firmly held by the ligaments, the fine spinal needle is pushed through it and on into the spinal canal (Figs. 63 and 65). Withdrawel of the stylet will reveal the escape of CSF (Fig. 64). CSF leakage can be rather slow with 25 and 26 gauge needles. Ideally CSF should continue to escape while the needle bevel is rotated slowly through 360°.

Should bone be contacted relatively superficially, it is probably the lamina of the vertebra. The needle or introducer must be withdrawn almost back to the skin and redirected (usually more cephalad). Because of their lack of rigidity it is not possible to redirect fine needles once they are engaged in ligament.

If bone is contacted deeply, it may be the anterior wall of the spinal canal. The stylet should be withdrawn and the needle retracted slowly while observing any leakage of CSF at the needle hub.

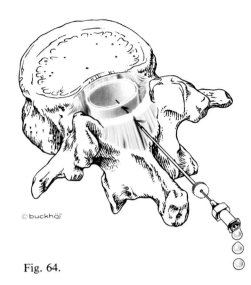

Fig. 64.

Fig. 63.

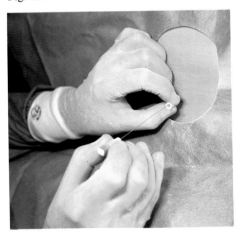

Fig. 65.

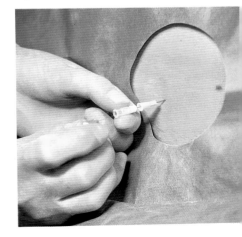

74

Injection of local anaesthetic

There is no point in injecting local anaesthetic if the needle tip is not unequivocally within the subarachnoid space, as shown by CSF leakage or easy aspiration of CSF with a syringe.

A syringe containing the calculated dose is attached to the needle hub and the plunger withdrawn a small distance to confirm the aspiration of CSF. The needle hub must be firmly held by the non-dominant hand during attachment of the syringe, aspiration and injection. Even a small movement may cause displacement of the needle tip.

A simple straightforward injection is all that is required. Barbotage is not feasible with small gauge needles and is unnecessary. Using a 5-ml syringe and a hyperbaric solution with dextrose, 1 ml every 5 s is the maximum rate of injection that can be made.

The needle is withdrawn and the patient turned into the desired position.

Fig. 66.

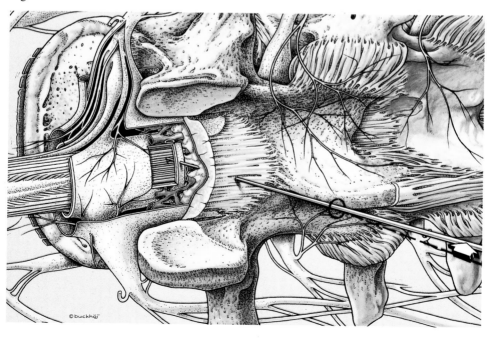

Factors affecting the spread of spinal anaesthesia

The number of spinal nerves that will be blocked following an intrathecal injection of local anaesthetic depends on many factors such as the dose and baricity of the solution and the posture of the patient. Though it is often believed that spinal anaesthesia is very predictable and easy to manipulate in regard to the height of block, Bier described it as "capricious", which it certainly is. Thus in spite of the best endeavours of the anaesthetist, considerable variations can and do occur and must be reckoned with.

1. Dosage would appear an obvious factor; increasing it would surely increase the spread. However, it has become clear that the relationship between dose and spread is not linear. Studies have shown only a minor additional spread when the dose of 0.5% hyperbaric bupivacaine is increased from 3 to 5 ml. In the range of 1-3 ml there are differences in the height of blockade, especially if the patient is sitting up for a few minutes after the injection, i.e. gravity is also affecting the spread.

2. Gravity can influence the height of spread but less than might be imagined, and only with hyperbaric solutions. Iso- and hypobaric solutions are virtually unaffected by posture as they mix easily and rapidly with CSF. Gravity only causes major differences in spread when it is maximal, i.e. when the patient's spine is vertical. Thus a small quantity, 1-1.5 ml, of hyperbaric solution will give a block confined to the sacral roots (a saddle block) if the patient is kept sitting up during and for several minutes after the injection. Using a larger volume, 3-4 ml, the difference between sitting up and lying down becomes much less marked.

Unilateral block can be obtained as long as the patient is kept in the lateral position. However, once the supine position is resumed, the block rapidly becomes bilateral.

The head-down position which should enhance cephalad spread, only increases the height of block to a small extent.

Changing posture involves movement of the spine and some authorities believe that this, and the associated movement of the spinal cord and spinal nerves within the subarachnoid space, can enhance the spread. Turning from a lateral position to the opposite lateral position has been claimed to considerably increase the height of block in patients undergoing Caesarean section.

3. Baricity. Even in the horizontal position, hyperbaric solutions in doses up to 3 ml produce higher blocks than isobaric or plain solutions. It may well be that the relative non-miscibility of glucose-containing solutions together with their hyperbaricity allows them to ascend into the thoracic part of the subarachnoid space, with gravity assisting the movement of drug in the natural curves of the spine.

4. Late pregnancy. Though a satisfactory direct comparison of spinal anaesthesia in late pregnancy and in the non-pregnant state is difficult if not impossible, there is clinical evidence to suggest that spinal blockade achieves higher levels in late pregnancy than at other times, and very high blocks may be encountered.

Factors affecting duration of spinal anaesthesia

1. Drug and dosage. The obvious way to control the duration of spinal block is to use a local anaesthetic with appropriate duration of effect. However, there is good evidence that duration is also closely related to dosage, the higher doses causing a longer block than the lower.

2. Vasoconstrictors such as epinephrine or phenylephrine have been shown to prolong spinal blockade, though there are differences in opinion regarding the clinical usefulness of this. The actual mode of action of vasoconstrictors within the subarachnoid space has not been defined, though it is clearly not identical with their mode of action at other sites.

There appears to be a difference in the prolongation according to the local anaesthetic drug used, the best effect being with tetracaine and the least with lidocaine and bupivacaine.

Vasoconstrictors appear to be able to cause very prolonged block (>8 h) in some patients, but their action is unpredictable in an individual.

If used, the recommended dosage is epinephrine 0.1 mg (0.1 ml of 1:1.000 solution) or phenylephrine 1 mg.

Failure of spinal blockade

This may be a partial failure, i.e. inability to reach a sufficiently high blockade, or a total failure in which little or no nerve block is apparent after 15-20 min.

Partial failure may be due to inadequate dosage but is more likely it is due to the wide individual variations that occur with spinal anaesthesia.

Total failure to produce a demonstrable nerve block does occur and will raise the issue of whether the local anaesthetic drug has deteriorated in the ampoule or there has been a problem during the sterilising process. Neither of these possibilities is very likely however. Given that local anaesthetic in adequate dose injected into the CSF **must** produce multiple spinal nerve block, one is left with the inescapable conclusion that during the injection the needle tip was **not** in the subarachnoid space. This could be due to slight movement during the injection, or the bevel of the needle being only partially inserted through the dura etc.

Whether the failure is partial or total, the anaesthetist should have a pre-arranged contingency plan. If the block has "missed" one or two dermatomes, this might be made good with a subcutaneous infiltration at the incision or the IV injection of a short acting opioid. If the failure is total, then there may have to be recourse to a general anaesthesia. Each patient will present an individual problem with a variety of solutions.

Complications

Hypotension

Widespread sympathetic blockade can cause a reduction in peripheral resistance due to vasodilatation. Because the venous capacitance is also increased, any impediment to venous return (e.g. head-up posture or caval occlusion) will cause a fall in cardiac output.

Hypotension may also be contributed to by hypovolaemia or caval occlusion, both of which require a degree of vasoconstriction to maintain a normal arterial pressure.

Sudden severe hypotension during spinal block in a conscious patient is usually due to vaso-vagal fainting. This is accompanied by pallor, bradycardia, nausea and vomiting and sweating. Patients may suffer a transient vagal cardiac arrest and can develop signs of coronary insufficiency. Consciousness will be lost during this period of arrest. This type of hypotension is not seen in patients given a concomitant general anaesthetic. Although a general anaesthetic enhances the hypotensive effects of spinal block, the decrease in arterial pressure is not precipitate and not accompanied by vagal activity with a marked bradycardia.

Treatment

If posture or caval occlusion are thought to be factors, the patient should be repostured without delay, e.g. left lateral and head down.

Because vasodilatation is the trigger to most hypotensive episodes, it is logical to give a vasopressor (see p. 28) which will usually act rapidly and effectively. Overdosage causing **hyper**tension is to be avoided. In late pregnancy the effect of vasopressors on uterine blood flow is often feared, but an adverse effect on the foetus is unlikely if overshoot hypertension is avoided, whereas prolonged hypotension will be deleterious to the foetus.

Fluids are of use if there is evidence of hypovolaemia, but they should be backed up with vasopressors if the arterial pressure is not rapidly restored.

Atropine may be used for severe bradycardia, but vasopressors with both α- and β-receptor activity, e.g. ephedrine, will increase the heart rate satisfactorily by themselves.

Total spinal anaesthesia

If by accident an excessive amount of local anaesthetic is injected into the subarachnoid space a high or total spinal anaesthetic will ensue. This will involve widespread paralysis with respiratory arrest, severe hypotension and, if there is substantial cranial spread, unconsciousness. All these will appear within a few minutes of the injection.

Treatment is by artificial ventilation and vasopressor support of the circulation. Though alarming, total spinal block can be effectively treated if the diagnosis is made promptly.

Neurological damage
See p. 31.

Headache
Post-lumbar puncture headache can be severely debilitating. It is due to leakage of CSF through puncture hole (caused by the needle) in the dura and arachnoid mater. Thus the size of the hole is important and this will depend upon the size of the needle, the direction of the bevel and whether or not mutiple holes were made in the dura. It, also seems to depend upon the patients age, younger patients being more affected than older ones.

The headache has distinct clinical features, being clearly related to posture, in that it is worst when sitting and standing and relieved by lying down. It usually starts on the first postoperative day but may be delayed until the third day. Untreated it may take several days to disappear.

Treatment
Oral analgesics can be used if the headache is not severe, but more aggressive treatment is needed if it persists or is clearly incapacitating the patient. This involves the use of a "blood patch" i.e. the epidural injection of the patients own blood. An epidural needle is inserted into the same or an adjacent interveterbral space as was used for the spinal anaesthetic. 10-15 ml of the patients blood is withdrawn and injected (without addition of an anti-coagulant) into the epidural space, using strict aseptic precautions.

This causes an immediate increase in CSF pressure (with relief to the headache) and stops further CSF leakage. The injected blood will clot and remain in the epidural space for several days. If after treatment the headache recurs the blood patch may be repeated.

Epidural blockade

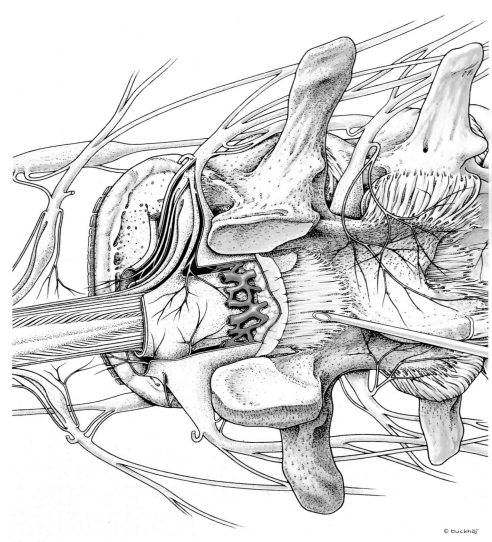

Fig. 67.

The epidural space lies within the spinal canal, outside the spinal dura mater. Local anaesthetic injected into the epidural space will spread both up and down the spinal canal, blocking the spinal nerves as they run from the spinal cord to their respective intervertebral foramina.

All modalities of nerve function will be affected by epidural block, namely motor, sensory and autonomic. However, it is possible to produce a differential block by adjustment of the concentration of local anaesthetic. Unlike spinal anaesthesia, when the local anaesthesia mixes with, and diffuses in, the cerebrospinal fluid, in epidural anaesthesia the local anaesthetic must spread by volume displacement. It is often assumed that local anaesthetic escapes from the epidural space through the intervertebral foraminae and that epidural injections are therefore unpredictable in their spread due to this leakage. For both anatomical and practical reasons, however, it is best to think of the epidural space as a closed space from which lateral escape does not occur or is very limited (Fig. 68).

Fig. 68.
1. Arachnoid mater
2. Subdural space
3. Dura mater
4. Periosteum
5. Ligamentum flavum
6. Pia mater
7. Subarachnoid space
8. Epidural space
9. Dorsal root ganglion
10. Periosteum
11. Posterior longitudinal ligament

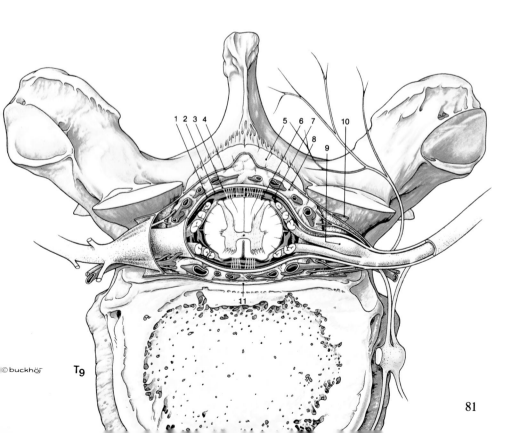

© buckhöj   T9

81

Anatomy

The spinal column in which the spinal canal runs is made up of seven cervical, twelfth thoracic, five lumbar and five (fused) sacral vertebrae (Fig. 69). These vary in their size, shape and strength depending upon the stress put upon them by the upright position. Thus the cervical vertebrae are the smallest and allow the greatest movement, while the lumbar are thick and robust with only limited movement (Fig. 70).

All vertebrae have a common structure, consisting of a vertebral body anteriorly and an arch of bone posteriorly, surrounding the spinal canal. The arch consists of two pedicles anteriorly and two laminae posteriorly. At the junction of a pedicle and a lamina is the transverse process. Where the laminae meet is the spinous process.

The spinous processes vary in regard to their caudal angulation, being almost horizontal except in the mid-thoracic region, where the angulation is most marked. This is of importance when attempting to locate the epidural space between T3 and T9.

The sacral vertebrae are fused together to form the sacrum, but the epidural space can still be entered through the sacral hiatus.

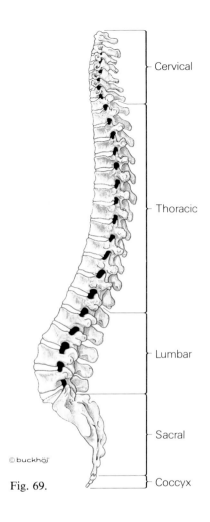

© buckhöj

Fig. 69.

Cervical

Thoracic

Lumbar

Sacral

Coccyx

Fig. 70.

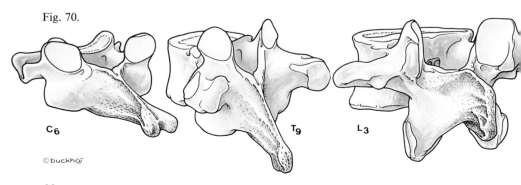

C_6

T_9

L_3

© buckhöj

82

Adjacent vertebrae are joined by the intervertebral discs and by the spinal ligaments. While the laminae and spinal processes are joined by ligaments, the pedicles are not. The gaps between the pedicles form the spinal foramina, through which the spinal nerves leave the spinal canal.

To reach the epidural space, the needle must pass through the supraspinous ligament, the intraspinous ligament and finally the ligamentum flavum, which joins adjacent laminae and is the thickest and toughest of the ligaments (Fig. 71).

The epidural space theoretically extends from the foramen magnum to the coccyx (Fig. 59). The spinal dura mater runs from the foramen magnum and ends around the first or second sacral vertebra. Although usually considered as a single layer of connective tissue, the spinal dura is a two-layered structure, the outer layer of which is closely applied to the wall of the spinal canal covering the bones, the discs and the ligaments which make up the canal (Fig. 68). This layer is often considered to be periosteum, but it not only covers bone but also ligaments and is easily stripped from them (unlike periosteum). In the cervical region the two layers are adherent from C1-C3.

The spinal cord runs from the brain to the level of L1/L2, while the inner layer of the dura mater ends at S1/S2 (Fig. 59).

Apart from spinal nerves, the epidural space contains fat, and blood vessels running to and from the vertebrae, the spinal cord, the meninges and the spinal nerves.

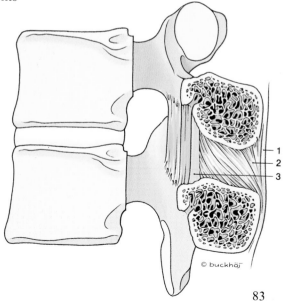

Fig. 71.
1. Supraspinous ligament
2. Interspinous ligament
3. Ligamentum flavum

The epidural space can be entered anywhere in its length from the C3-4 interspace to the sacral hiatus at S4-5. Because the spinal cord ends at L1-2, the commonest point of entry is the lower lumbar region. The nerves of the cauda equina all enter the epidural space at the termination of the internal layer of spinal dura, i.e. at S1-2. Thus a lumbar approach can easily block all the sacral nerves while at the same time local anaesthetic can ascend to block the thoracic segments.

However, there are advantages to entering the epidural space at levels other than the lumbar in order to produce discrete bands of anaesthesia at the appropriate height. Thus epidural block can be cervical, thoracic, lumbar or sacral (caudal).

Spinal nerves supply specific dermatomes in the body and different upper levels of block are required for different operations as follows:

Upper abdominal	T5-6
Lower abdominal	T8-9
Lower limb	T12
Perineal	S1
Bladder	T10
Kidney	T8

The autonomic nervous system

The preganglionic sympathetic nerves arise from the 14 spinal segments from T1-L2, while the sacral parasympathetics derive from S2-4 (Fig. 72). Widespread blockade of autonomic nerves can have profound physiological effects.

Fig. 72.
1. Pharyngeal plexus.
2. Superior vagal ganglion.
3. Inferior vagal ganglion.
4. Celiac ganglion.
5. Celiac plexus.
6. Inferior mesenteric ganglion.
7. Superior hypogastric plexus.
8. Inferior hypogastric plexus.
9. Superior cervical ganglion.
10. Middle cervical ganglion.
11. Stellate ganglion.
12. Superior mesenteric ganglion.

Parasympathetic

Sympathetic

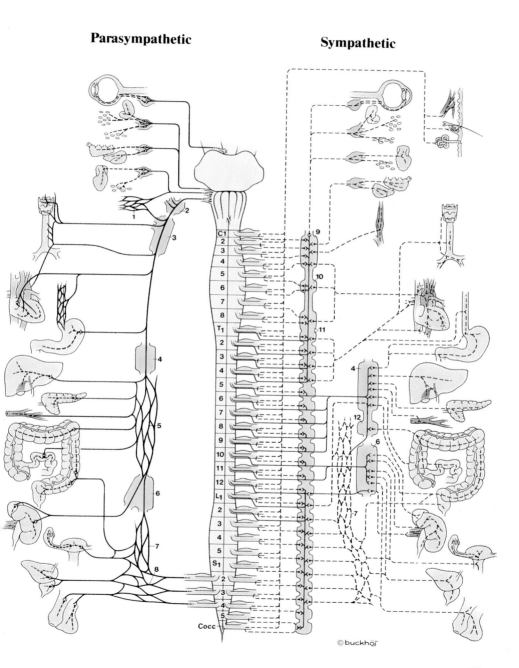

© buckhöj

Equipment

Because the spinal canal is being entered and subarachnoid puncture can occur accidentally, it is essential that all aseptic and antiseptic precautions are taken. The anaesthetist should wear sterile rubber gloves and work with a sterile pack. Because catheter techniques are commonly used to extend the duration of the block, Tuohy needles (16 or 18 gauge) with a Huber point are the most popular.

The pack should also contain:

1. Syringes. If the loss of resistance technique is being used, the plunger of the syringe should move easily and without resistance within the barrel.
2. Needles. Large for drawing up fluid from ampoules and small for intradermal injection.
3. Ampoules of local anaesthetic and saline.
4. Stylet for making a hole in the skin before inserting the Tuohy needle.
5. Swabs, lotion pot and sterile drapes for preparing the skin.
6. Epidural catheter and bacterial filter.

Patient position

1. Lateral with spine fully flexed (Fig. 73)
2. Sitting with feet on stool and bending forward.

Patient preparation

Epidural blocks should only be performed where full anaesthetic facilities are available. A standard anaesthetic machine and all resuscitative equipment and drugs must be at hand. All anaesthetists performing epidural block should be able to diagnose acute generalised toxicity and total spinal anaesthesia quickly should they occur. Treatment is simple and effective, but must be applied without delay (see p. 27 and 94).

An intravenous infusion should be set up as the first step. Blood pressure and heart rate should be recorded and many would insist that the electrocardiogram be displayed. The patient should be positioned as described above.

The patient's back is prepared with an appropriate antiseptic solution as for a surgical operation, and sterile drapes applied (Fig. 73).

Fig. 73.

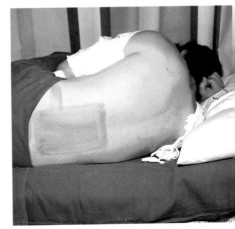

Lumbar epidural blockade

Landmarks

The bony landmarks are palpated (Fig. 73). The iliac is felt at the level of the L4 vertebra (Fig. 74).

The L2-L3 and L3-L4 interspaces are those most commonly used.

Needle insertion

An intradermal wheal is raised with local anaesthetic exactly over the chosen interspace. Subcutaneous infiltration may also be used.

A large sharp needle or a stylet is then pushed through the skin to make a hole and allow easy insertion of the epidural needle.

Holding the skin firmly over the spinous processes with the index and middle fingers of one hand the epidural needle is inserted in the midline at right angles to the skin. The skin should not be allowed to move, otherwise the needle may be inserted too far laterally.

The needle is advanced until it is firmly engaged in the interspinous ligament. It now has to penetrate the ligamentum flavum to reach the epidural space (Fig. 71). The stylet is withdrawn.

Fig. 74. Courtesy of Astra.

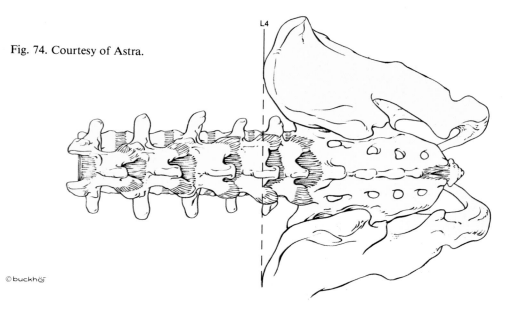

© buckhöj

Identification of the epidural space

Loss of resistance technique

The commonest method used is the loss of resistance technique. There are many variations of this technique, some using the hands and others mechanical aids.

A syringe containing saline or air is attached to the needle lying in the interspinous ligament. Injection will be found to be difficult or impossible. The most difficult part of the technique to learn is the control of the advancing needle, which must not penetrate the epidural space beyond the needle bevel. The position of the hands and fingers on the needle and syringe are critical.

The index finger of the non-injecting hand may be held firmly against the patient's back to act as a resistance to sudden forward movement. The thumb and middle finger hold the needle hub (Fig. 75).

Alternatively the dorsum on the non-injecting hand is placed on the patient's back and the fingers can be turned back to hold the needle at its hub. The hand thus acts as an "opponens" to the advancing syringe and needle.

This may even be exaggerated so that the hand grasps the lower end of the syringe.

Where advancement of the needle is relatively easy, continuous pressure on the syringe plunger can be used, care being taken that the needle is pushed through the ligamentum flavum slowly and without a sudden forward movement, which could lead to penetration of the dura mater.

As the needle is advanced, pressure is maintained on the plunger, noting the increased resistance of the ligamentum flavum. At the moment of entering the epidural space, saline or air can be injected with great ease.

The flow of fluid (or air) from the syringe as the needle enters the epidural space pushes the dura away from the needle point (Fig. 76).

Fig. 75.

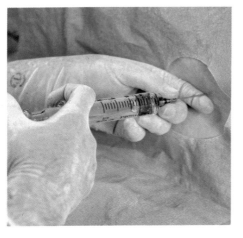

Fig. 76.

© buckhöj

When a blunter needle is preferred or the ligaments are difficult to penetrate, then an intermittent technique can be used. Both hands push on the needle in a controlled way and the resistance to injection is tested after every millimetre of advancement.

Mechanical aids include the Macintosh balloon, an intravenous infusion and a springloaded (Evans) syringe. These allow two-handed advancement of the needle (which is helped by a winged needle) and the immediate identification of the epidural space as the resistance to injection disappears.

"Hanging drop" technique

The negative pressure that is often found within the epidural space is the basis for the "hanging drop" technique. A winged needle can be used and it is advanced with both hands. A drop of fluid is placed at the end of the needle after engaging the interspinous ligament (Fig. 77). When the ligamentum flavum is penetrated the drop of fluid is sucked into the epidural space, and correct identification of the space can be confirmed by injection of fluid or air without resistance. Unfortunately a negative pressure cannot always be demonstrated and many anaesthetists feel this method is less reliable than the loss of resistance technique.

Catheter technique

If a prolonged nerve block is required, a plastic catheter can be introduced through the needle (Fig. 78) so that repeated injections can be made to provide a continuous epidural block for the duration of surgery and, if required, into the postoperative period. This, of course, also applies to epidural block used for relief of pain in labour.

Fig. 77.

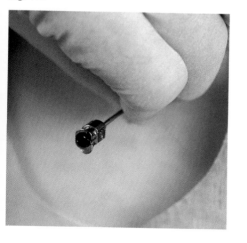

Fig. 78.

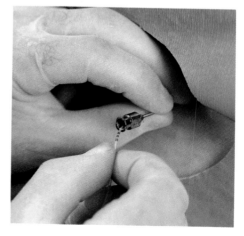

A plastic catheter with appropriate (5 cm) distance markings is used. It is passed through the needle and into the epidural space.

The catheter is rolled in one hand to prevent it falling into an unsterile area.

A slight resistance is felt as the catheter passes through the tip of the needle, when the second distance mark will just be visible at the hub (Fig. 79).

By turning the needle, the Huber point can be directed cephalad or caudad. The catheter can therefore be advanced in either direction.

About 5 cm of catheter is advanced into the epidural space, when the third distance mark will be at or near the needle hub.

The needle is then withdrawn carefully without removing the catheter, which is gently pushed forward as the needle is being retracted.

The needle is completely removed from the patient.

There are several different designs of catheter available. Some have a single terminal opening, while others have up to three lateral holes. Some are supplied with a stylet. Most are somewhat rigid at their tip and can penetrate the thin wall of an epidural vein. All are provided with a means of connecting the proximal end of the catheter to a syringe.

A bacterial filter can be attached to the end of the catheter so that all fluid injected is sterile.

Water-resistant strapping is used to keep the catheter in place.

All injections can now be made near the patient's head (Fig. 80).

Fig. 79.

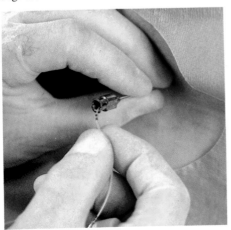

Fig. 80.

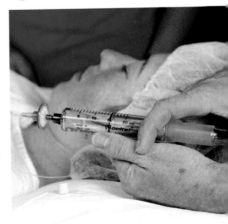

Drugs and dose

Test dose

Before injecting the chosen dose of drug, many anaesthetists prefer to inject a small test dose to eliminate the possibility of the needle or catheter being either in a vein, or within the subarachnoid space.

The amount of drug used as a test dose and the time allowed must be adequate to show the effects of incorrect placement. Thus 4-5 ml of drug injected into the subarachnoid space and left for 5 min will give an easily detected spinal block, whereas 2 ml left for 2 min might well not do so. 2 ml of a hyperbaric spinal solution will show most quickly that a subarachnoid injection has been made, but will have very little effect in the epidural space, unlike say 5 ml of 2% lidocaine or 0.5% bupivacaine, which may produce a block over several spinal segments. If the needle or catheter is lying within a vein, even 5 ml may be insufficient to cause systemic effects unless epinephrine (0.1 mg, i.e. 0.1 ml of 1:1.000 solution) is added and the heart rate and arterial pressure are measured before and after injection. **It is important that if a test dose is used, a negative result should not be taken as absolute proof of correct placement.** Care must still be taken while injecting the main dose. If a test dose has been given through the needle, a further test dose should be given after insertion of the catheter.

Main dose

Many drugs can be used for epidural block (Table 4 p. 24). Because of the size and thickness of the coverings of the spinal nerves, drugs must be used in high concentration for complete nerve blockade, though weaker solutions may be used for pain relief; this is especially so when the pain is mediated through autonomic nerves, as with the pain of uterine contractions during labour.

The volume to be used (Table 5) will depend upon the required height of blockade and the general condition of the patient.

Table 5.
Volumes used for lumbar epidural blockade

Operation	Volume (ml)
Lower abdominal	15-20
Upper abdominal	15-25
Lower limb & perineal	10-15
Pain relief in labour	6-10
Postoperative pain relief	6-10

A common misconception is that the spread within the epidural space is linear related to the volume injected, i.e. 20 ml will involve twice as many spinal nerves as 10 ml. This is not so, because of the variability in the potential volume of the epidural space at different levels in the spinal column, and to the erratic spread of the first 5-10 ml of injectate. The last 10 ml of a 20-ml injection is likely to "fill out" the space where local anaesthetic has already reached, rather than spread to a higher level. Thus a 20-ml injection will produce a more profound and longer lasting nerve block, but will be only a few segments higher, than a 10-ml injection. There is no evidence that posture plays any part in the spread of local anaesthetic solutions in the epidural space.

The simplest approach to dosage is to plan on injecting rather more than is thought necessary to block nerves to the required level. Thus failure to achieve an adequate height will be greatly reduced and more prolonged blockade will result. Unduly high blocks are uncommon and if properly managed will cause little upset to patients unless they are either very old or very ill. With a catheter, dosage can be varied at will according to the response to the initial injection.

Because the total dose of the drug is likely to cause toxic effects if given rapidly into an epidural vein, **it is important to inject slowly** (10 ml/min) even though the test dose gave a negative result. An alternative approach is to inject the local anaesthetic in small aliquots, e.g. 5 ml every 5 min until the necessary height of blockade is achieved.

Complications

Misplacement of needle or catheter

The anaesthetist must ensure that the needle tip or the catheter is in the epidural space. If the catheter has been incorrectly inserted and does not lie within the spinal canal, then no nerve block will result from the injection of local anaesthetic. This possibility must be entertained if there is no evidence of a nerve block within 15-20 min. The most likely position of the catheter in such a case is the sacrospinalis muscle, lateral to the spinous process. This can occur particularly in obese patients. The anaesthetist can be misled by the ease of injection, since a loss of resistance can occur when the needle deviates laterally from the interspinous ligament and reaches the muscular compartment.

Dural tap

Most dural taps are due to an uncontrolled sudden forward movement of the needle as the ligamentum flavum is penetrated. Dural tap will be diagnosed by removing the syringe and observing cerebrospinal fluid (CSF) escaping from the needle. CSF may be distinguished from the fluid used in the syringe by its temperature or by the presence of glucose. If the subarachnoid space has been entered the escape of CSF through the large bore needle is usually so copious that there is little doubt as to the true position of the needle. A spinal headache is liable to result (see p.79).

Intravenous placement

Penetration of an epidural vein by the needle is easy to detect as blood flows freely from the needle hub. In such a case the needle must be withdrawn and the procedure repeated at the same or an adjacent vertebral interspace.

Intravascular placement of a catheter, however, may be much more difficult to diagnose. Catheters advanced through the needle can penetrate vein walls and this must be checked before injecting large quantities of local anaesthetic. Simple aspiration may reveal the intravenous placement (Fig. 81) but this is not totally reliable as the negative pressure applied may suck the vein wall against the end of the catheter and obstruct it. It is best to lower the protruding end below the patient's spine and allow any blood to escape by gravity. If frank blood is seen, the catheter must be removed and reinserted. If blood-stained fluid is seen, the catheter or needle may or may not be in a vein. A test dose as described above may then be useful in determining the location of the catheter or needle.

Hypotension

Widespread sympathetic blockade can cause a reduction in peripheral resistance due to vasodilatation. Because the venous capacitance is also increased, any impediment to venous return (e.g. head-up legs-down posture or caval occlusion) will cause a fall in cardiac output.

Hypotension may also be contributed to by hypovolaemia or caval occlusion, both of which require a degree of vasoconstriction to maintain a normal arterial pressure.

Sudden severe hypotension during epidural block in a conscious patient is usually due to vaso-vagal fainting. This is accompanied by pallor, bradycardia, nausea, vomiting and sweating. Patients may suffer a transient vagal cardiac arrest and can develop signs of coronary insufficiency. Consciousness will be lost during this period of arrest. This type of hypotension is not seen in patients given a concomitant general anaesthetic. Although a general anaesthetic enhances the hypotensive effects of an epidural block, the decrease in arterial pressure is not precipitate and not accompanied by vagal activity with marked bradycardia.

Fig. 81

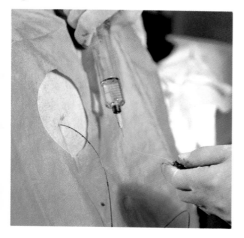

Treatment

If posture or caval occlusion is thought to be a factor, the patient should be re-postured without delay, e.g. left lateral and head down.

Because vasodilatation is the trigger to most hypotensive episodes, it is logical to give a vasopressor (see p. 28) which will usually act rapidly and effectively. Over-dosage causing **hyper**tension is to be avoided. In late pregnancy the effect of vasopressors on uterine blood flow is often feared, but an adverse effect on the foetus is unlikely if overshoot hyperten-sion is avoided, whereas prolonged hypo-tension will be deleterious to the foetus.

Fluids are of use if there is evidence of hy-povolaemia, but they should be backed up with vasopressors if the arterial pressure is not rapidly restored.

Atropine may be used for severe brady-cardia, but vasopressors with both α- and β-receptor activity, e.g. ephedrine, will increase the heart rate satisfactorily by themselves.

Acute generalised toxicity

Because epidural block often requires large amounts of local anaesthetic, toxic reactions can occur and constant vigi-lance is required. The use of aspiration before injection and a test dose (provided epinephrine is added) will help prevent these reactions. Slow injection of the main dose is also essential. The symp-toms, signs and treatment of toxic reac-tions are described on p. 25-27.

Total spinal anaesthesia

If by accident an excessive amount of local anaesthetic is injected into the sub-arachnoid space, a high or total spinal anaesthetic will ensue. This will involve widespread paralysis with respiratory arrest, severe hypotension and, if there is substantial cranial spread, unconscious-ness. All these will appear within a few minutes of the injection.

Treatment is by artificial ventilation and vasopressor support of the circulation. Though alarming, total spinal block can be effectively treated if the diagnosis is made promptly.

Neurological damage

See p. 31.

Headache

See p. 79.

Suggested further reading

Introduction

Covino BG & Vassallo HG (1976). Local Anesthetics: Mechanisms of action and clinical use. Grune & Stratton, New York.

Arthur GR. Wildsmith JAW & Tucker GT (1987). Pharmacology of local anaesthetic drugs. In Principles & Practice of Regional Anaesthesia. Eds. Wildsmith JAW & Armitage EN. Churchill Livingstone, Edinburgh, p. 22.

Charlton JE (1987). The management of regional anaesthesia. In Principles & Practice of Regional Anaesthesia. Eds. Wildsmith JAW & Armitage EN. Churchill Livingstone, Edinburgh, p. 37.

Pither CE, Ford DJ, Raj PP (1984). Peripheral nerve stimulation with insulated and uninsulated needles: efficacy and characteristics. Regional Anaesthesia 9. 42.

Brachial plexus block

Winnie AP (1984). Plexus Anesthesia I, Perivascular Techniques of Brachial Plexus Block. JH Schultz A/S, Copenhagen.

Lower limb

Winnie AP, Ramamurthy S, Durrani Z (1973). The inguinal perivascular technic of lumbar plexus anesthesia: the 3 in 1 block. Anesthesia & Analgesia 52, 989.

Moore DC (1979). Regional block (4th edition) Charles C Thomas, Springfield.

IV Regional

Duggan J, McKeown DW & Scott DB (1984). Venous pressures in intravanous regional anesthesia. Regional Anesthesia 9. 70.

Lee A, McKeown DW, Wildsmith JAW (1986). Clinical comparison of equipotent doses of bupivacaine and prilocaine in intravenous regional anesthesia. Regional Anesthesia 11. 102.

Intercostal nerve block

Katz J, Renck H (1987). Handbook of Thoraco - abdominal Nerve Block. Mediglobe SA, Fribourg.

Moore DC (1975). Intercostal nerve block for post-operative somatic pain following surgery of the thorax and upper abdomen. Brit J Anaesth 47. 284.

Spinal anaesthesia

Lee JA, Atkinson R & Watt MJ (1985). Lumbar Puncture & Spinal Analgesia (5th edition). Churchill Living-stone, Edinburgh.

Lund PC (1971). Principles and Practice of Spinal Anesthesia. Charles C. Thomas, Springfield, Illinois.

Cousins MJ & Bridenbaugh PO (1987). Neural Blockade (2nd Edition) Lippincott, Philadelphia.

Epidural blockade

Bromage PR (1978). Epidural Analgesia. Saunders Co. Philadelphia.

Covino BG & Scott DB (1985). Handbook of Epidural Analgesia & Anaesthesia. JH Schultz A/S, Copenhagen.

Index